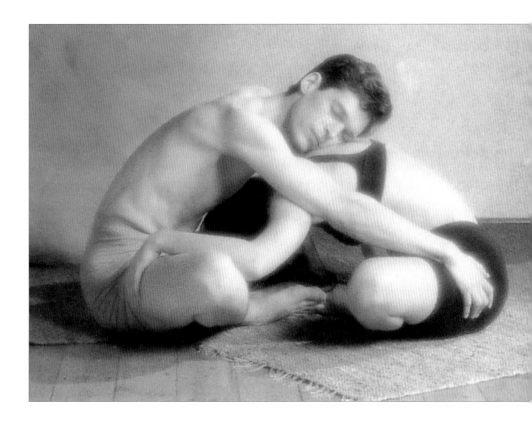

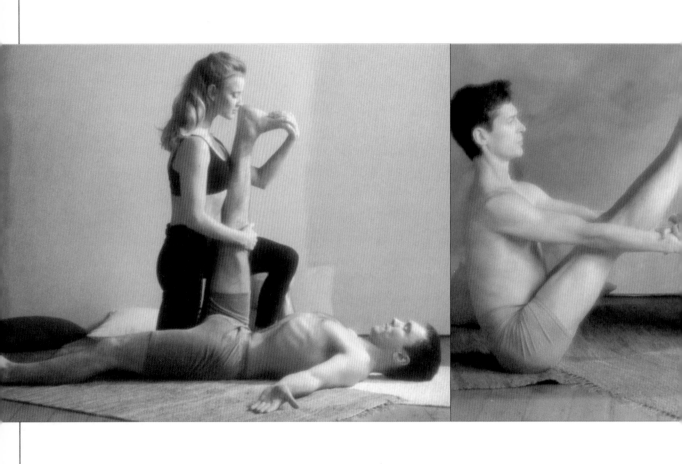

THE ART OF SENSUAL YOGA

A STEP-BY-STEP GUIDE FOR COUPLES

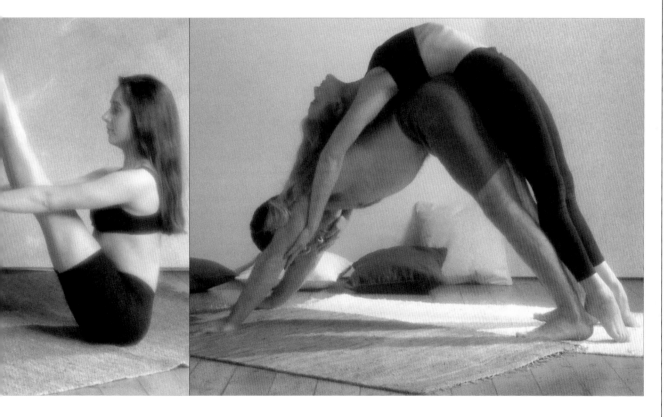

CONNIE AND ROBERT DUNNE KIRBY
WITH GERALDINE ROSS

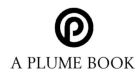

A PLUME BOOK

PLUME
Published by the Penguin Group
Penguin Books USA Inc., 375 Hudson Street,
New York, New York 10014, U.S.A.
Penguin Books Ltd, 27 Wrights Lane,
London W8 5TZ, England
Penguin Books Australia Ltd, Ringwood,
Victoria, Australia
Penguin Books Canada Ltd., 10 Alcorn Avenue,
Toronto, Ontario, Canada M4V 3B2
Penguin Books (N.Z.) Ltd, 182–190 Wairau Road,
Auckland 10, New Zealand

Penguin Books Ltd, Registered Offices:
Harmondsworth, Middlesex, England

Published by Plume, an imprint of Dutton Signet, a division of
Penguin Books USA Inc. First published in Great Britain as *Yoga for
Lovers* by Smith Gryphon Limited.

First Plume printing, February 1997
10 9 8 7 6 5 4 3 2 1

Designed by Hammond Hammond, London
Edited by Helen Armitage
Photographed by Peter Shoesmith

ISBN 0-452-27820-1

CIP data is available.

Printed and bound in Spain by Grafos SA, Barcelona

**Although great care has been taken to ensure the
safe practice of *The Art of Sensual Yoga,* the authors
and publishers can accept no responsibility for any
injury or ill-effect from any of the poses. Couples
should exercise within the limits of each partner.**

CONTENTS

THE AUTHORS

CONNIE DUNNE KIRBY was born in Ireland, educated in England and lived and worked in China, where she studied acupuncture in Nanjing. She has an acupuncture clinic in central London and uses the treatment in her therapeutic work with couples. As a yoga practitioner for some 15 years she has liaised closely with Geraldine Ross to devise the series of movements featured in *The Art of Sensual Yoga*, many of which she encourages her clients to adopt in their daily routines.

ROBERT DUNNE KIRBY is an agent with the international Sheil Land literary agency. Coming rather late to yoga, he was stunned by the positive effects it had on their relationship and how its regular practice not only promoted their personal well-being but also that of other couples working together to develop deeper and more caring relationships. He, with his partner Connie, through their own personal practice, have refined and modified ancient yogic postures specifically to meet their own needs and those of other couples in the 1990s.

GERALDINE ROSS began practicing yoga 20 years ago to get back into shape after the birth of her first child. She is a qualified Hatha Yoga teacher, with clients that include Amnesty International, Touche Ross, John Lewis, Lingfield Health Clubs and Coopers & Lybrand. She quickly became aware that the physical and spiritual aspects of yoga could have profound effects on relationships between couples and has been working with this in mind to develop new postures.

ACKNOWLEDGEMENTS

The authors would personally like to thank the following people for their help and inspiration: Carol-Anne Adams, Nadia Adorni, Andrulla, Chicky, Kim Jacobs, Graham, Ivan Ross, Jamie Roberts, Kate O'Connor, Luke O'Sullivan, Martin, Sean Ross and Simon Trewin. Special thanks go to the Smith Gryphon crew: our publisher, Robert Smith; editor, Helen Armitage; designer, Roger Hammond and photographer, Peter Shoesmith. Finally we'd like to express our heartfelt thanks to our models: Edward Clark, Desiree Kongerød, Martin McDougall and Philippa Vasadari.

The authors and publishers would like to thank Nice Irma's, London, for props used throughout this book.

A Note from the Authors

THE ART OF SENSUAL YOGA is a new and unique form of yoga practice, which expertly tailors the ancient principles of yoga to the specific needs of couples living in the 1990s. This is a major breakthrough. Until now yoga has been perceived as a solitary process, in which the individual, through the practice of meditation, exercise and breathing, achieves harmony and well-being. But this innovative technique, evolved over a period of some 20 years, has been developed in response to the growing demand from couples to work together to improve the quality of their lives and relationships.

All you need to practice *The Art of Sensual Yoga* is a little time and a comfortable space. Anyone can do it. You don't need special equipment or clothes – just a loving partner! The yoga postures adapted for *The Art of Sensual Yoga* stretch and tone every part of the body, both internally and externally, keeping all systems fit and healthy. They are designed to release physical and mental tension in order to set free natural resources of energy.

With an accessible text and evocative photographs, *The Art of Sensual Yoga* is an easy to follow, step-by-step system of enjoyable exercise, which can help people not only to feel well in themselves but also to benefit from healthier relationships with each other. By improving physical and mental health, regular practice of *The Art of Sensual Yoga* increases the ability to deal with the challenge to all partnerships that stressful, distracted late 20th-century life-styles can bring.

To the many hundreds of couples whose relationships have blossomed through the practice of The Art of Sensual Yoga *and without whom this book would not have been written*

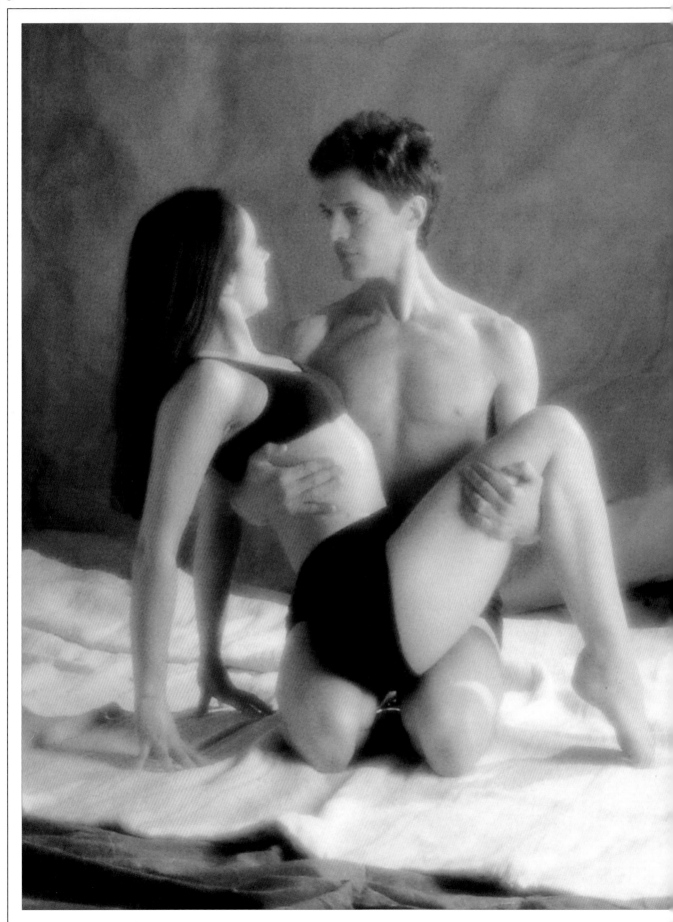

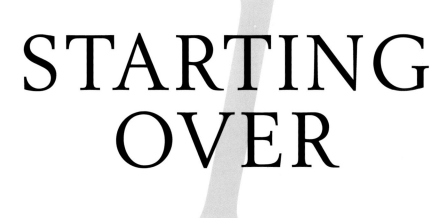

STARTING OVER

O N A PSYCHOLOGICAL LEVEL our deepest need as men and women is to overcome our separateness; to leave the prison of our aloneness. This desire for interpersonal fusion is our most powerful struggle. It is our most fundamental passion. It is the force that keeps the human race together!

To love somebody is not just a strong feeling – it is a decision, it is a judgement, it is a promise.

As human beings we are gifted with reason, with self-awareness and an awareness of others, of our past and of the possibilities for our future. This awareness of ourselves as a separate entity, our consciousness of our aloneness and separateness arouses our fears; it is, indeed, the source of all anxiety.

People, of all ages and cultures, are confronted, then, by the question of how to overcome separateness, how to achieve union. There are many answers to the one question. Some of us seek for the answer in the oblivion supplied by drugs and alcohol, others through the constant repetition of sexual union, others still through the comfort and union of conformity. And many of us through the state of being in love.

In relationships, if we project our positive images on to each other at the same time, we have that seemingly perfect state known as being in love, a state of mutual fascination. As a couple we then declare that we are 'in love with each other' and are firmly convinced that we have now found the ultimate relationship.

There is much to be said for falling in love. Most of us can probably remember the first time we were in love, and what unexpected and powerful emotions were released. To have the experience of falling in love is to become open to matters of the heart in a wonderful way. It can be the prelude to a valuable expansion of personality and emotional life. It is also an important experience because it brings the sexes together and initiates relationships. Whether this leads to happy or unhappy consequences, undoubtedly life is kept moving in this way.

The fact is, however, that relationships founded exclusively on the being-in-love state can never last. The harsh truth that the condition of being in love cannot endure the stress of everyday life is not what we want to hear. We decide to go on looking for the perfect man or woman. Because of this many of us prefer to go from one person to another, always seeking the ultimate relationship, leaving it when the projections wear off and the in-loveness ends. It is obvious that with such shallow roots no real, permanent love can develop. To be capable of real love signals maturity, with realistic expectations of the other person. It means accepting responsibility for our own happiness or unhappiness, and neither expecting our partner to make us happy nor blaming them for our own bad moods and frustrations.

Love between two people is possible only if we communicate with each other from the heart of our existence. In this central experience is human reality based, and here there is aliveness, here the basis for love. Love, experienced thus, is a constant challenge, not a resting-place but a moving, growing, working together. Whether there is harmony or conflict, joy or sadness is secondary to the fundamental fact that we experience each other from the essence of our being, that we are at one with each other – by being at one with, rather than fleeing, ourselves. There is a simple proof for the presence of love: the depth of the relationship, and the vitality and strength in each person concerned. This is the fruit by which love is recognized.

The Art of Sensual Yoga uses the principles of yoga to guide lovers to develop mature, loving relationships that endure. The first step to take is to become aware that love is an art, just as living is an art; if we want to learn how to love we must proceed in the same way we would if we wanted to learn any other art, say music, painting, carpentry, or the practice of medicine or engineering. The process of learning can be divided conveniently into two parts: one, the mastery of the theory; the other, the mastery of the practice. *The Art of Sensual Yoga* is a guide to the mastery of the practice.

Why do we, in our culture, try so rarely to learn this art, given our obvious failures at it? Could it be because, in spite of the deep-seated craving for love, almost everything else is considered to be more important? Success, prestige, money, power – almost all our energy is used to gain knowledge of how to achieve these aims, and almost none to perfecting the art of loving.

As with the practice of any art, *The Art of Sensual Yoga* has certain general requirements: a willingness to develop openness, strength and humility, to use patience, care and self-knowledge. Its practice has been inspired by many workshops conducted over the past 20 years. Time and again it was observed that when stu-

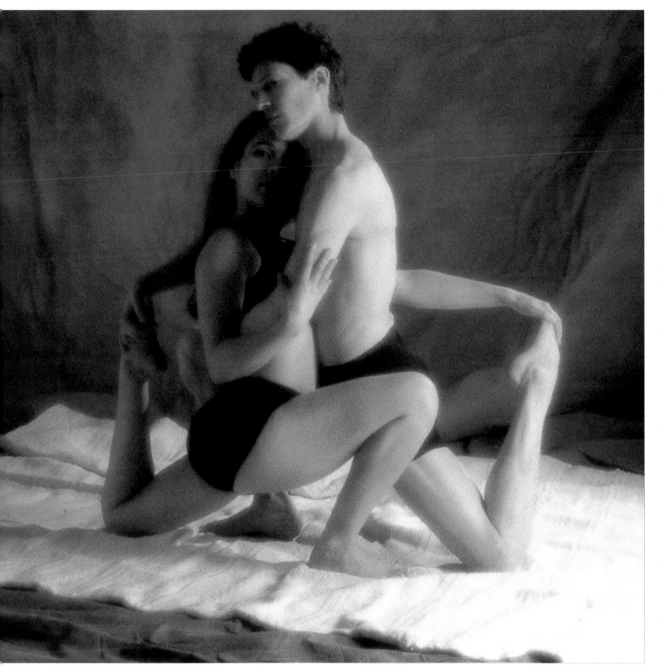

On a psychological level our deepest need is to overcome our separateness

dents worked together, guiding and supporting each other into and out of yoga postures, the energy of the class changed. Close physical contact, combined with breathing, stretching and lifting, helped students explore relationships in a deeper and more meaningful way.

The Art of Sensual Yoga is based firmly on personal experience: the feedback and inspiration of participating couples, from all walks of life, many of whom say how much it has improved both the physical and emotional aspects of their relation-

ships. Experience clearly shows that, with just a small investment of time, *The Art of Sensual Yoga* can help to make the life-style changes that are so vital to the maintenance of all intimate relationships. The word yoga literally means 'union'. Now, with this dynamic approach to yoga exercise and relaxation, countless couples are growing closer and uniting more deeply and more joyfully in their partnerships.

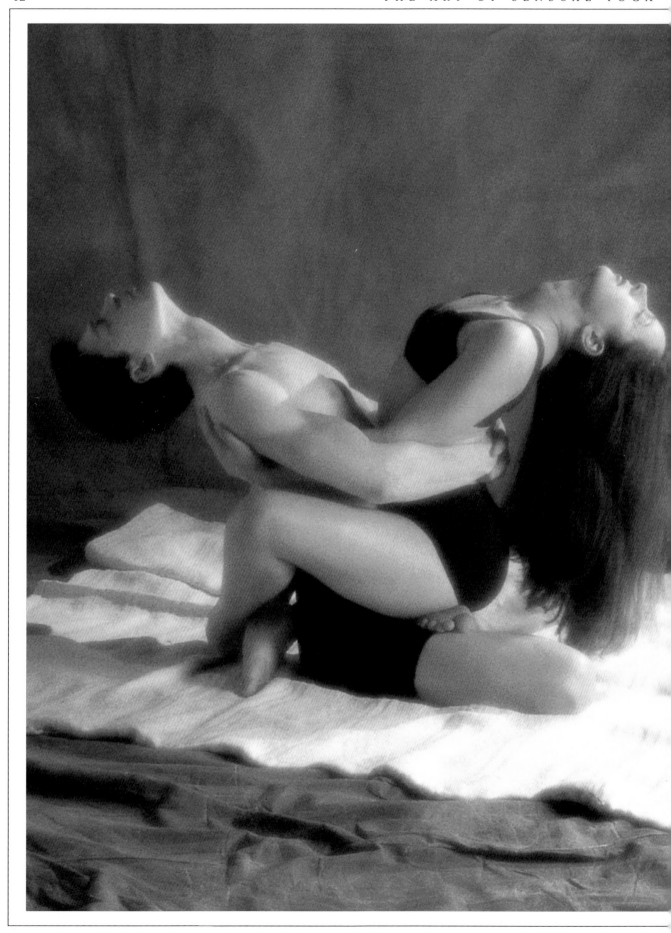

WHAT IS YOGA?

The Art of Sensual Yoga is based on postures – called asanas in Sanskrit, the ancient Indo-Germanic literary language of India – that are inspired by the art of yoga, a complete science of life, developed several thousand years ago in India. Yoga is older than Christianity and one of the oldest systems of personal development in the world. The philosophy behind it is based on an understanding of the nature of humanity and our needs. Its practice involves an integration of mind, body and soul. Balance is the key.

Over the past 30 years yoga (from the Sanskrit *yuj*, 'to bind together') has become increasingly popular in the West as a way of stimulating vitality, enhancing good health and the general ability to relax. Its practice is continually evolving, as each new generation reinterprets its principles in accordance with its needs. This new yoga for the 21st century is practical, straightforward and achievable by anyone with a basic level of fitness. It has been successfully tried and tested in hundreds of workshops and practical sessions.

PHYSICAL BENEFITS

Medical research shows that yoga can do much to:
• Relieve high blood pressure
• Help such diverse ailments as arthritis, arteriosclerosis, chronic fatigue, asthma, varicose veins and heart conditions
• Increase lung capacity and respiration
• Reduce body weight
• Improve ability to resist stress
• Decrease cholesterol and blood-sugar levels
• Stabilize and restore the body's natural systems

EMOTIONAL BENEFITS

Couples report the following emotional benefits:
• General improvement in stress management
• Greater openness in communication
• Deeper mutual care, trust and understanding
• Increased sensual awareness
• Enhanced libido

GENERAL POINTS

DO'S

• If you have a basic level of fitness, you can do the sequences in this book.
• Go slowly, even if you have been doing other forms of physical exercise.
• Every practice should ideally be preceded by the warm-up sequences in chapter 2, 'Loving Yoga'. Practice the sequences in the order in which they are presented in each chapter.
• Wear loose clothing; whatever feels comfortable.
• Work on a non-slip surface with bare feet.
• Rest when your body is tired. Your stamina will increase as you practice regularly.
• Relax your muscles and never force your body into a stretch.
• Go into each movement on the out-breath and then breathe normally. Do not hold your breath as this causes tension and strain.
• Come out of the positions with as much care as you go into them.

DONT'S

• Do not practice immediately after eating.
• If you have severe backache, don't start stretching without consulting your doctor. Although exercise may well form part of the treatment, you should first obtain a proper diagnosis.
• Do not practice in direct sunlight or in a cold room.
• To avoid injury, never force the body beyond its capacity.
• It is not advisable to begin yoga while pregnant, as there are so many physiological changes that take place within the body during that time.

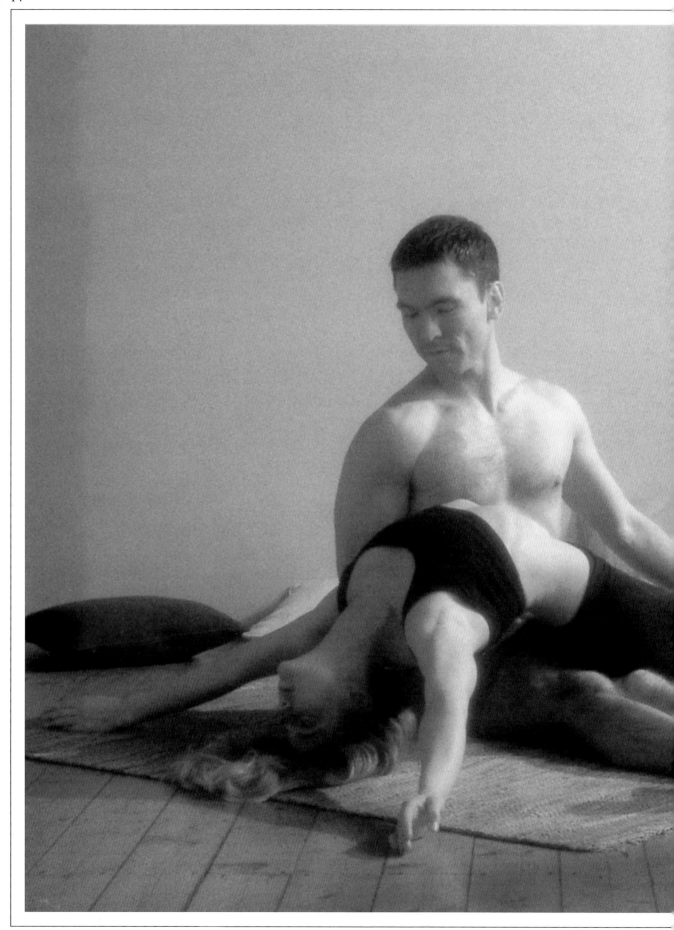

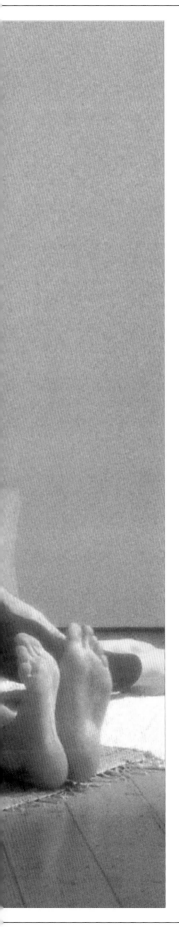

LOVING YOGA

CREATING THE SPACE

FIRST CREATE A NURTURING environment for yourselves, especially if you have both had a busy and stressful day. Take a shower and be comfortable afterwards in what you do or don't wear. So as not to disturb yourselves once you have begun exercising, you may wish to light some candles, assemble some cushions and play some relaxing music. Whatever else you do, you should make sure the room is warm.

Before starting the first sequence of movements in each chapter, just sit quietly, cross-legged and facing each other, and breathe softly but deeply. Hands should rest on the knees, palms upward. See if you and your partner can breathe at the same pace, without strain – getting slowly into the same quiet space.

Desire is like the changing seasons. It waits, stirs, excites and finally fulfills.

1. BEING

PHYSICAL EFFECTS

Simply sitting cross-legged helps to release stiffness in the hips, a problem for many of us in the West given our life-style, which involves little squatting or sitting on the floor.

The twisting action is excellent for toning and stretching the spine, liver, kidneys and intestines. The shoulders and upper chest are stretched too.

In the final part of the sequence the chest is opened, and the spine is stretched. This helps to improve lung capacity significantly.

This sequence will allow you both to feel much more open and revitalized. Your energy should become calmer. Ideally you should begin to feel comfortable just being together.

EMOTIONAL REFLECTIONS

These simple twists gently stimulate the liver – the seat of anger. If you feel a sense of irritation, release and let go of any negative feelings.

MEDITATION
I open myself to a calm state of being

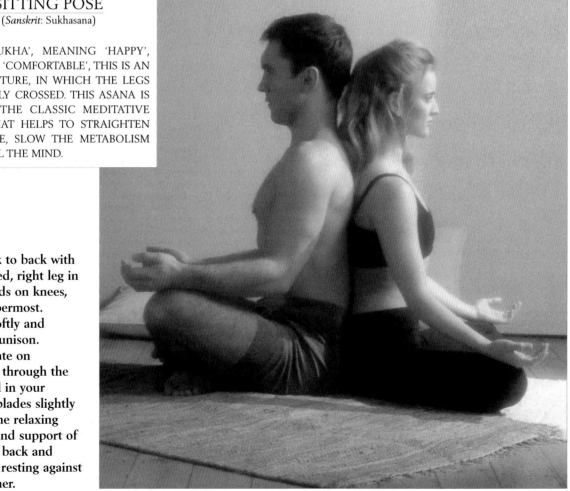

SITTING POSE
(*Sanskrit*: Sukhasana)

FROM 'SUKHA', MEANING 'HAPPY', 'EASY' OR 'COMFORTABLE', THIS IS AN EASY POSTURE, IN WHICH THE LEGS ARE SIMPLY CROSSED. THIS ASANA IS ONE OF THE CLASSIC MEDITATIVE POSES THAT HELPS TO STRAIGHTEN THE SPINE, SLOW THE METABOLISM AND STILL THE MIND.

1. Sit back to back with legs crossed, right leg in front, hands on knees, palms uppermost. Breathe softly and deeply in unison. Concentrate on stretching through the spine. Pull in your shoulder-blades slightly and feel the relaxing pressure and support of your hips, back and shoulders resting against your partner.

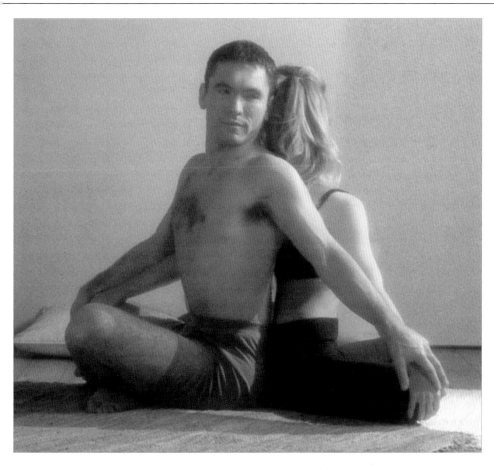

2. Reach behind, first with the left hand, for your partner's knee. This automatically twists the spine to the left, but remember to keep your back straight and shoulders back. Hold this twist for four to five breaths.

3. Return to the center, then twist to the right again by reaching back and placing your right hand on your partner's knee. Hold again for four to five breaths.

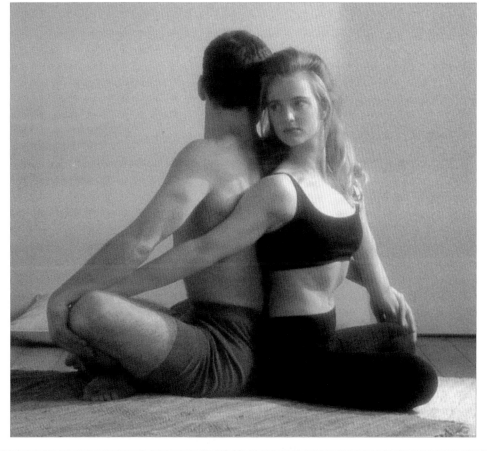

4. (right) Return to the center; one partner then leans forward from the hips. Bend forward as far as it is comfortable to go, keeping the buttocks firmly on the floor. Let your neck follow the line of your spine and take your hands to the side. The sitting partner then leans back, stretching over the hips and back of the other. Allow the chest to open and extend the head back, opening the neck and chest. Stretch the arms to the side, joining hands, palm to palm. Hold for four to five breaths.

5. Return to the center, reverse the position and hold.

6. (right) Return to the center, recross your legs and repeat the entire sequence from stage one.

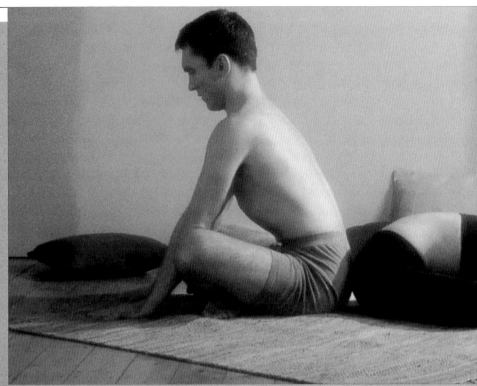

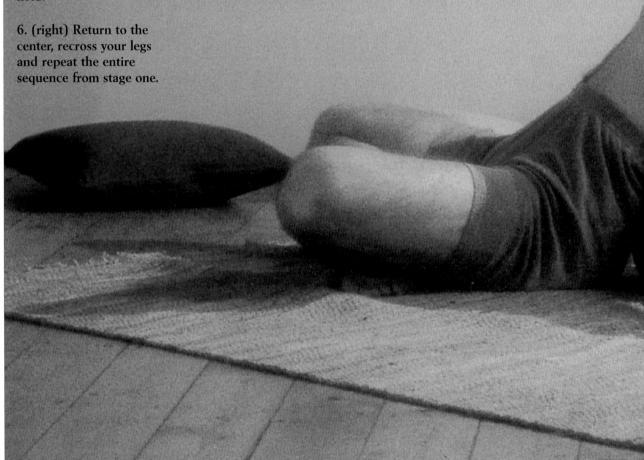

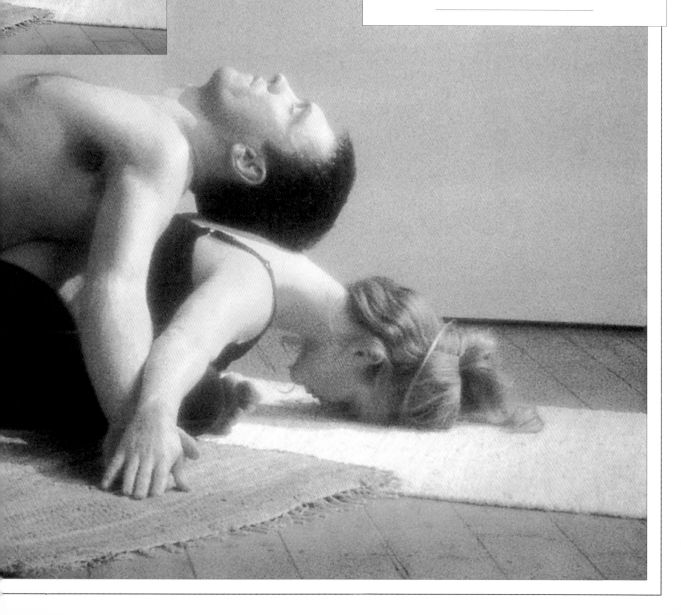

HELPFUL HINTS

• IF YOUR HIPS feel uncomfortable sitting on the floor, use a cushion to support the buttocks.

• SEE IF YOU can breathe together as you make the movements. Breathe out as you go into the posture and breathe in as you come out of it.

• REMEMBER TO KEEP the throat and jaw completely relaxed.

• IF YOU FIND the forward bends too strenuous, you can put your hands in front of you to support yourself and your partner. Similarly with the back bend, use your hands to give you extra support.

2. OPENING

PHYSICAL EFFECTS

This posture is wonderful for removing sluggishness as it tones the liver, spleen and pancreas. It also strengthens the intestines and all the abdominal organs. It helps to remove excess fat from the waist area, flexes the hips and removes strain in the lower back. Also, with the aid of your partner, the chest is opened and the shoulders and arms stretched.

In the final movements of the sequence any strain in the back is released by one partner pressing down gently on the upper shins and then stretching the legs away from the hips.

You will feel toned and released after completing this sequence – it really does help to remove the inner 'cobwebs'.

EMOTIONAL REFLECTIONS

The hips store emotional and sexual tension. They also carry the body in balance. In this sequence concentrate on letting go of the past and opening up to the future.

MEDITATION
I am ready to move on – I am open to the future

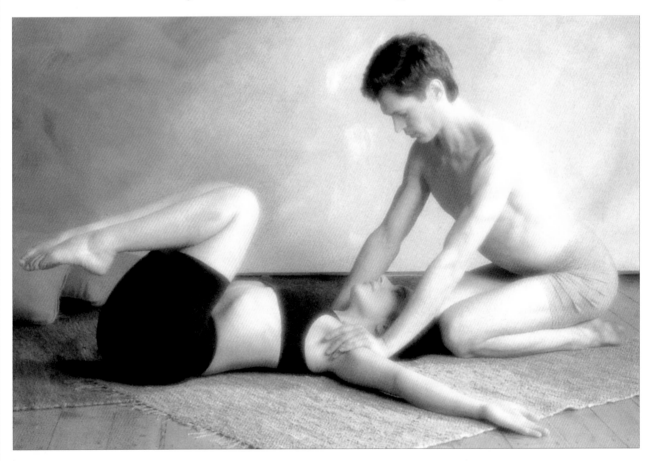

1. Lie back flat on the floor, lifting your knees to your chest. Your partner should sit on their heels, at your head, and press down gently on your shoulders. Stretch your arms to your side with the palms facing upward.

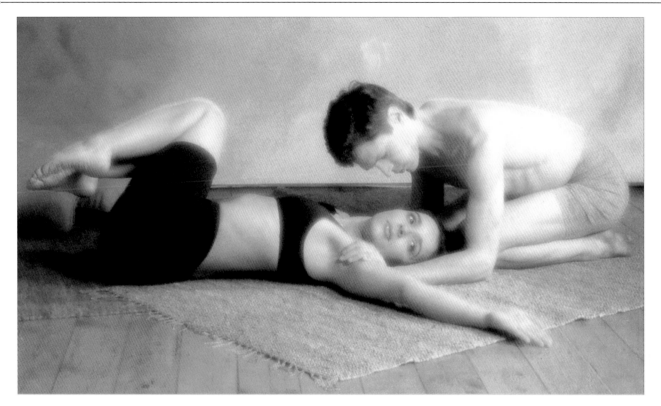

2. Keeping the knees and ankles together, slowly take them over towards the right armpit. The kneeling partner continues to press the shoulders down to maintain stability in the posture. Try to keep the bent knees off the floor and hold for four to five breaths.

3. (below) Return your knees to the center in a slow and controlled movement.

4. Then take your knees over to the left armpit and hold for four to five breaths.

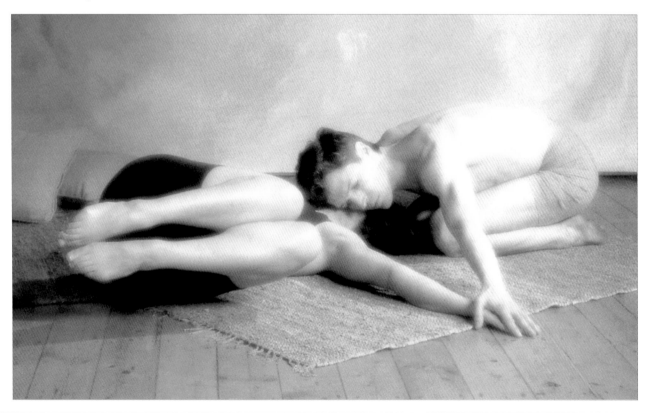

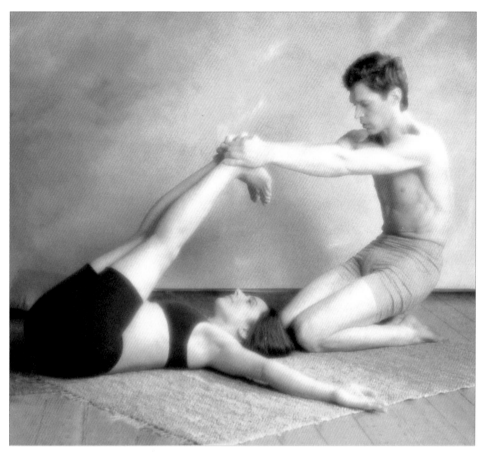

5. Return your knees to the center. The sitting partner reaches forward taking hold of your heels and extending your legs as far as they will comfortably go towards your head. Hold for four or five breaths.

6. Return your knees to the center and allow the sitting partner to push down on your shins to stretch the lower back. Change positions and repeat from stage one.

HELPFUL HINTS

• TRY TO KEEP the back flat on the floor, turning only from the hips.

• PERFORM THE MOVEMENT on the out-breath and release out of it on the in-breath.

• KEEP THE ARMS well stretched throughout.

• THROAT, JAW AND eyes should remain passive.

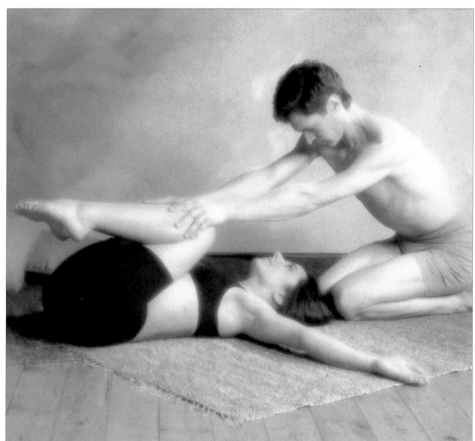

3. THE GATEWAY

PHYSICAL EFFECTS

In this posture you are using each other's bodies to help stabilize in the pose and to achieve the maximum stretch.

The pelvic area, abdominal muscles and organs are toned and stretched, and the sequence provides an excellent release for the spine. The intercostal muscles between the ribs are gently stretched, so breathing capacity improves.

You will begin to feel much more in tune with your partner in this pose as you support and stretch each other, releasing and breathing together.

EMOTIONAL REFLECTIONS

This sequence stimulates, in particular, the liver and heart. The heart is often considered the seat of love and security, joy and happiness.

MEDITATION
I give my heart to you

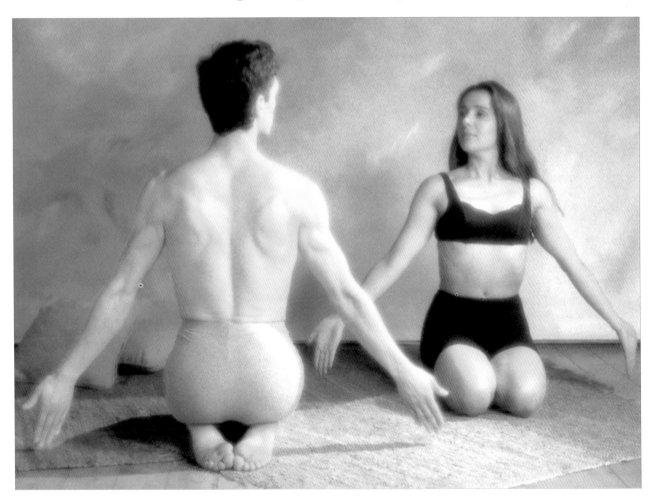

1. Sit on your heels, facing each other at a slight distance. You will gauge the space apart when you go into the third stage. Stretch out your arms to your sides, palms open. Keep your spine straight, shoulders back and chest open.

2. Come up on to your knees, with the thighs perpendicular to the floor, knees and feet together.

3. With an exhalation, extend your right leg to the side. Your inner foot should press against your partner's knee, and your right hand should reach out and rest on your partner's shoulder. Your left hand should rest on your hip. Stretch through the extended arms.

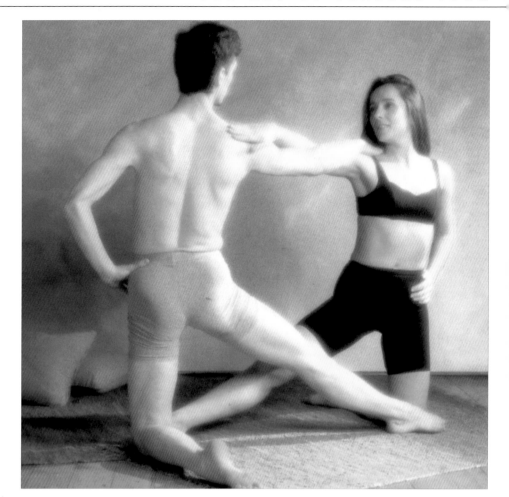

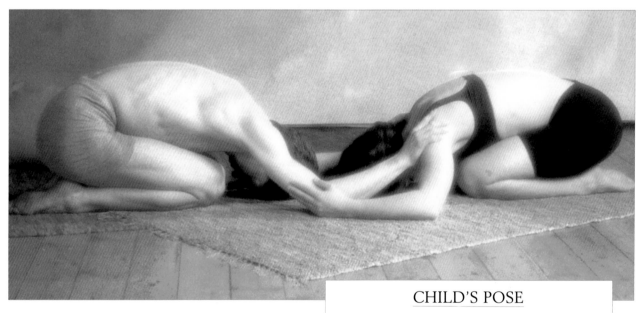

5. Return to the first-stage position and turn to face each other. Lean forward, resting on your heels, stretch your arms forward in CHILD'S POSE.

6. Turn around and repeat this sequence extending the opposite legs and arms.

CHILD'S POSE

THIS RELAXATION POSE IS USED TO NORMALIZE THE CIRCULATION AND TO GIVE A COUNTER-STRETCH TO THE SPINE. KNEEL DOWN AND SIT BACK ON YOUR FEET, HEELS POINTING UPWARD. PLACE YOUR FOREHEAD ON THE FLOOR, THEN BRING YOUR ARMS ALONGSIDE YOUR BODY, PALMS TURNED UPWARD.

4. With an exhalation, stretch the left arm up and catch your partner's elbow. At the same time place the back of the right hand on the top of the extended leg knee.

Stretch over towards each other. Keep the shoulders back, shoulder-blades tucked in and throat and jaw soft and relaxed.

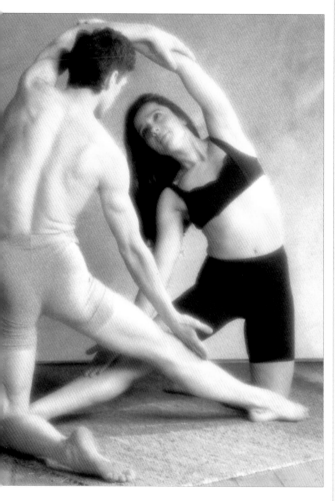

HELPFUL HINTS

• THIS SEQUENCE IS strong so take plenty of time going into it. Only stretch as far to the side as you feel comfortable with.

• COMPLETE THE EARLIER sequences before attempting this one.

• THE BREATHING IS important; keep it slow and deep. As you begin to go into the posture breathe out, and complete the pose on the inhalation.

• HOLD EACH POSTURE for four to five breaths.

Lifestyle choices

Much of this book covers the physical and emotional benefits of practicing yoga together. But as you work through the sequences, and as your yoga practice develops, you will find that you will become, subtly at first, more aware of your body, your relationship and your lifestyle in general. Initially this awareness is often detected in an increased sensitivity to what you put into your body – your diet.

In yoga, energy has three qualities, or Gunas, which exist in equilibrium. They are Sattva, Rajas and Tamas, which represent purity, the process of change, and darkness, respectively. These energies are manifest in all matter, and the philosophy behind them is similar to the Chinese principles of Yin and Yang: the two opposing, yet complimentary, sides of nature.

In any object – or situation – one quality is predominant. This is as much relevant to, say, an apple, as it is to a relationship. Thus on an apple tree some of the fruit is ripe (sattvic), some ripening (rajasic) and some overripe (tamasic). Similarly, a relationship can be a loving alliance between equal partners (sattvic), developing (rajasic) or destructive (tamasic).

Sattvic food is the purest diet. It nourishes the body, quiets the mind and increases the general flow of energy between them. Sattvic foods include cereals, wholemeal bread, fresh fruit and vegetables, pure fruit juices, milk, butter and cheese, nuts, seeds, honey and herb teas.

Hot, bitter, sour, dry or salty foods are rajasic. They destroy the mind–body equilibrium by feeding the body at the expense of the mind. They are over-stimulating, making the mind restless, and include sharp spices and stimulants, such as coffee, tea and chocolate.

Tasmic items lower energy levels, destroy body cells and disturb the mind. These include meat, alcohol, tobacco, fermented foods and stale or overripe substances. Overeating is also regarded as tasmic.

Yoga teaches us the benefit of equilibrium: passive awareness and take in nothing to excess. This represents one of the greatest yogic teachings: follow the Middle Way.

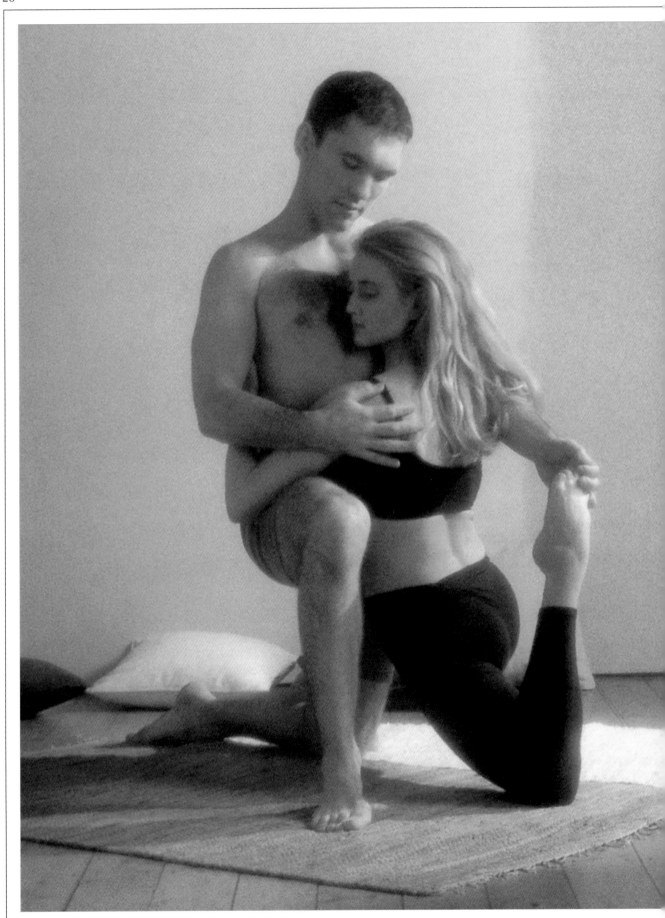

GETTING TOGETHER

RELATIONSHIPS BETWEEN COUPLES should be mutually rewarding; ideally each partner's weaknesses are balanced by the other's strengths. As individuals we are drawn to partners who can satisfy areas of our lives in which we feel deficient, or we may look for someone who is strong and on whom we can depend. Unfortunately this comfortable state of affairs may stagnate the relationship as there is no need for either to strive for individual self-awareness. If the relationship breaks up, the subsequent feelings can be similar to a bereavement; each partner may be left unable to cope without the assistance of their 'other half'.

Falling in love is a natural and beautiful experience, and a life that has not known this experience is impoverished.

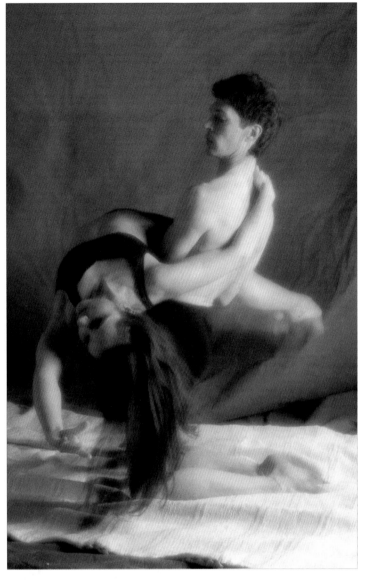

The Art of Sensual Yoga **can take relationships to new heights of caring and sharing**

The ideal relationship, however, is one built on love, respect and honesty, where both partners are able to remain whole and yet be enhanced by the union. Sadly, such a large part of our lives today is defined by a materialistic, commercial and mass-media orientated culture. Nearly every aspect of our lives seems to be packaged in one sense or another, and this contributes little to a sensitive and caring relationship between people. In order for our loving relationships to flourish and grow we need to take time to be close to each other, to be peaceful and gain experience of each other.

Many of us are turning away from the rat race and taking responsibility for our own lives and well-being; we are looking at the ancient arts of healing and exercise that are all-embracing and work on a deeper level than many modern forms of exercise. Of these yoga is certainly among the most popular. It works at so many different levels, not only the physical but the mental, emotional and spiritual as well.

The Art of Sensual Yoga is a tool, or an instrument, to help guide us to deeper loving relationships. To understand what its practice is all about we need to experience it for ourselves. At first glance it seems to be little more than a series of strange physical postures, which can keep the body lean and flexible. But, in time, anyone who continues practice will become aware of a subtle change in their approach to life. Through persistently toning and relaxing the body and stilling the mind, and working in this way while supporting each other, we begin to glimpse a state of the inner peace that is our true nature.

The yoga-based exercises in this chapter, when practiced carefully and with due diligence, are a prayer to any relationship. They can enhance the attraction between a couple and take the partnership to new heights of caring and sharing. There is no better way to iron out problems with your relationship than to work your bodies together. Holding and stretching one another can say so much more than words. Then, when speech comes, it does so from a less superficial, more loving space.

The sequences that follow are a little more challenging and the supporting role of the partner more integral to achieving the full movement. They are suitable for any period of the day, whenever you have some time to be together without interruption. They will feel very good and relaxing, and you'll both feel, inevitably, more together.

There are many ways of being together – going for a walk, playing tennis, or having a meal – each of which is fine. But by adding the practice of *The Art of Sensual Yoga* to your joint itinerary, all the other ways of relating and spending time together will be immeasurably enhanced.

1. EXPRESSION

PHYSICAL EFFECTS

Sitting cross-legged releases stiffness in the hips. The spine is toned, and the abdominal organs are gently stretched on both sides. The intercostal muscles are also stretched.

This posture is invigorating, and the counter-posture at the end of the sequence balances the energy and releases any strain in the back.

EMOTIONAL REFLECTIONS

Emotional blockages are often contained in the chest muscles; by stretching these muscles feelings can become released. If you experience strong emotions arising, try not to suppress them. Let them find expression.

MEDITATION

I give myself to my emotions and allow them full expression

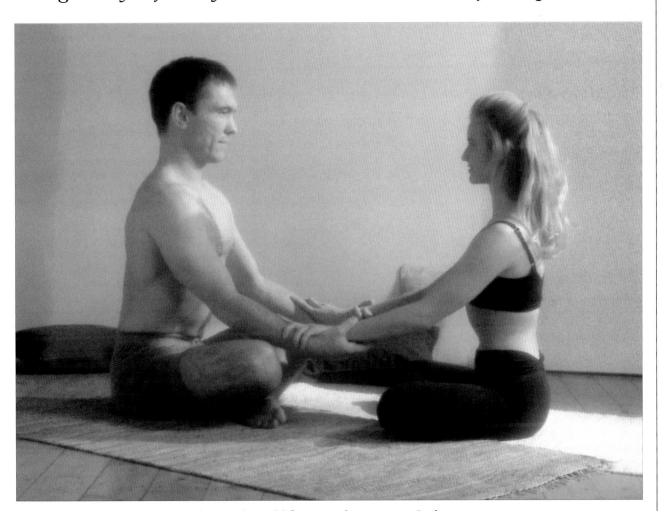

1. Face each other in the SITTING POSE and take hold of your partner's wrists. Let your arms hang loosely, and remember to keep your back straight and lift through your spine. Keep your shoulder-blades tucked in. Breathe softly and allow your body to relax into the position. Seek out any areas of tension and release with the out-breath.

2. Twist your upper bodies in the same direction, and each raise one arm, still linked at the wrists, up over your heads. Lower the other arm, again still linked at the wrists, so that the action of the elbow pressing into the knee helps to rotate the spine. Hold for four to five breaths.

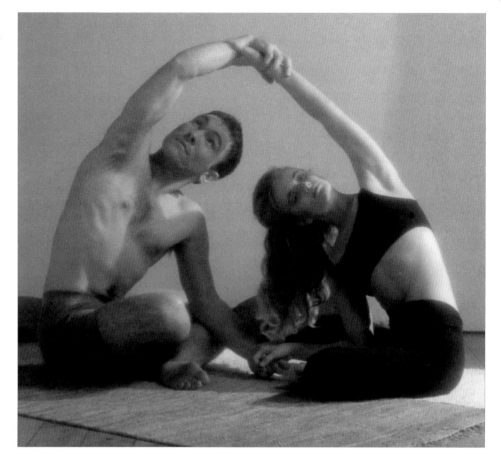

3. (left) Release back to center and reverse the twist, again holding for four to five breaths.

4. This sequence should be repeated after recrossing the legs with the other leg in front.

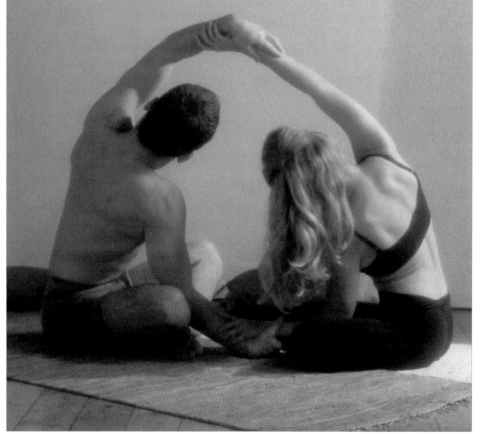

5. (opposite) One partner turns from the hips and places their head on the other's knee; the other partner relaxes over the back of the lower partner. Hold for four to five breaths and then come back up and reverse with the other partner on top.

HELPFUL HINTS

• IF THE HIPS are stiff and you find the cross-legged position uncomfortable, sit on a cushion or folded blanket.

• WHEN YOU DO the upper-body twist, feel your ribs stretching away from the waist.

• IT IS IMPORTANT that the shoulder-blades are tucked in to allow the collar-bones to lift.

• THE THROAT, as usual, should remain soft.

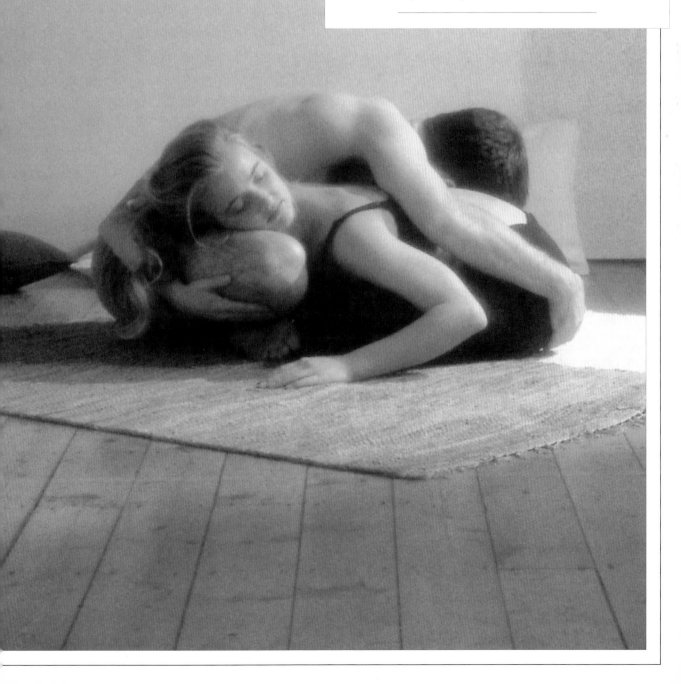

2. MOVING FORWARD

PHYSICAL EFFECTS
This posture stretches the legs and tones the ankles. It also helps release stiffness in the hips. The chest is opened, and the lower back is toned and relaxed as the bent leg is taken over to one side. This posture is particularly good for lower-back strain and for problems associated with sciatica.

Postures working on releasing stiffness in the hips can have a profound effect on general well-being. A great number of acupuncture points pass through the hips, so those channels are opened with these stretches.

EMOTIONAL REFLECTIONS
Stiff hips and legs inhibit our ability to move forward emotionally, which is most often expressed as a feeling of treading water, of standing still in life and not developing one's true potential. Release the stiffness and allow your dreams and ambitions to flow.

MEDITATION
I have taken the first step, and the path is clear

1. Lie down on your back with the arms fully extended to the side, palms upward. Stretch out both legs and sink your heels, hips, chest, shoulders and head down into the floor. Stretch into your heels, and pull your toes forward as far as is comfortable. Keep your throat soft and jaw relaxed.

2. The supporting partner takes hold of the right leg at the knee and toe and lifts gently upwards, raising the leg as far as it will go without strain. Hold for four to five breaths.

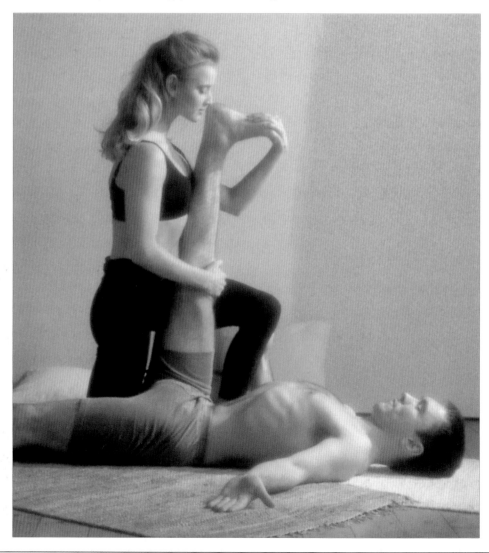

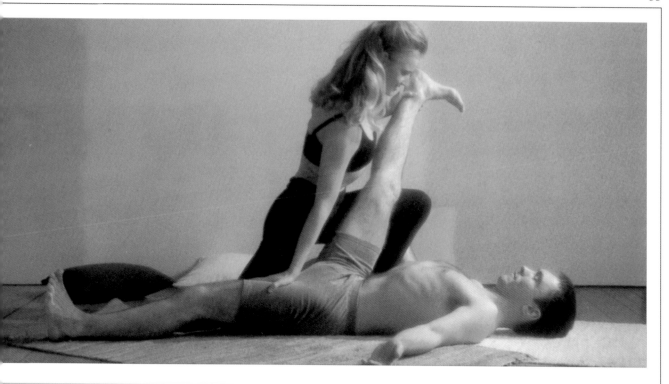

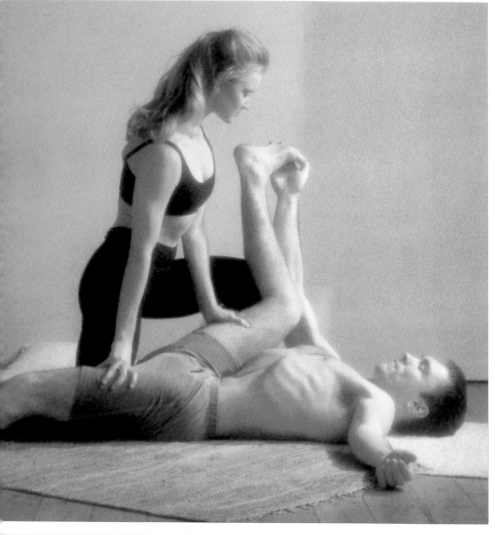

3. The right leg is then lowered to its side – again go only as far as it is comfortable. Increase the stretch by pressing firmly into the left thigh of the reclining partner and hold for four to five breaths. Take leg back to the center.

4. Bend the raised right leg at the knee and reach for the toe, pulling the foot down and taking the knee into the right armpit. Keep the shin vertical. Hold, keeping the lower leg stretched; the supporting partner then pushes the bent leg, aiming the knee towards the right armpit. Hold again for four to five breaths.

5. Place foot of the bent leg on the opposite knee. Supporting partner presses down on the right knee and shoulder, stretching the hip. Hold for four to five breaths.

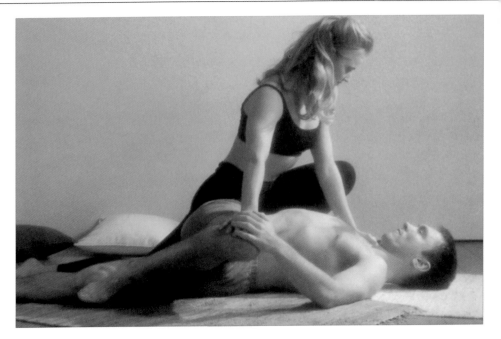

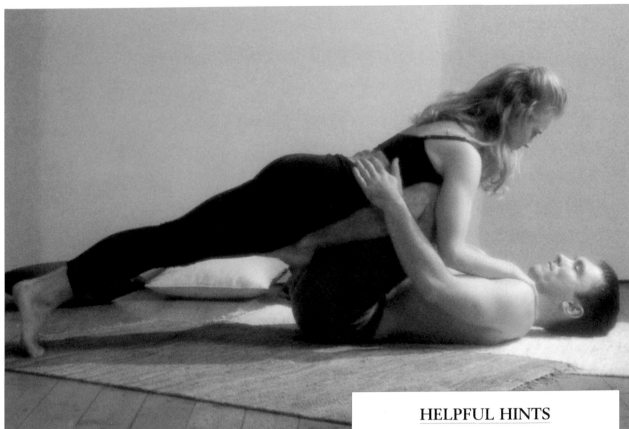

6. Repeat with the left leg, then bring both knees up to the chest. The other partner then lies on the knees, pressing down evenly with their body weight to release any lower-back strain.

7. Switch roles.

HELPFUL HINTS

• DON'T RUSH THESE movements, and beware of overstretching the legs and hips.

• BE CAUTIOUS IN using your full body weight in the counterpose. Be guided by your partner.

3. STRENGTHENING

PHYSICAL EFFECTS

This sequence is strong and difficult to hold, so it is an excellent one to do together, using each other's legs and arms as support.

The sequence can be most effective in calming gastric complaints, in toning the kidneys and in strengthening the lower back.

After completing the poses your whole body will feel warm and alive.

EMOTIONAL REFLECTIONS

Stress and anxiety can cause kidney problems. On an emotional level strengthening the kidneys and lower back can help to deal with the feeling of loss of determination, stamina and drive, to strengthen the will and to overcome anxiety and stress.

MEDITATION

I face life with strength and courage – I have all the support I need

1. Sit in COBBLER POSE **and support each other's arms. Make sure your toes are touching. Breathe deeply and relax.**

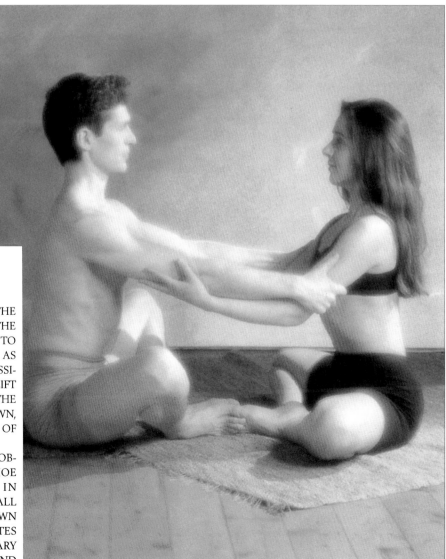

COBBLER POSE
(*Sanskrit*: Baddha Konasana)

SIT WITH THE SOLES OF THE FEET TOGETHER, SLIDING THE HEELS AS NEAR AS YOU CAN TO THE GROIN. TAKE THE KNEES AS CLOSE TO THE FLOOR AS POSSIBLE WITHOUT STRAIN AND LIFT THROUGH THE SPINE. KEEP THE SHOULDERS BACK AND DOWN, AND THE SIDE AND BACK OF THE NECK EXTENDED.

THIS IS CALLED THE COBBLER POSE BECAUSE SHOE MENDERS AND MAKERS IN INDIA SIT IN THIS POSITION ALL DAY LONG. IT IS WELL KNOWN THAT THE POSE STIMULATES THE KIDNEYS, AND URINARY DISEASES ARE RARELY FOUND AMONG INDIAN COBBLERS.

2. Bring your own knees together, lean back slightly, holding each other's hands to maintain balance. Keep the lower back, ribs and chest lifting and neck extended.

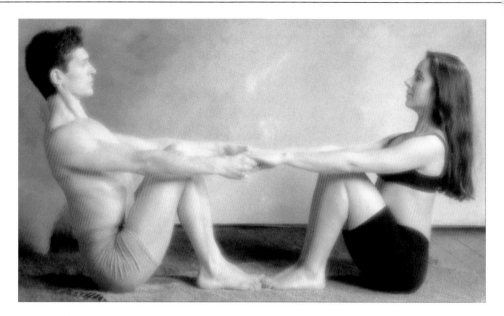

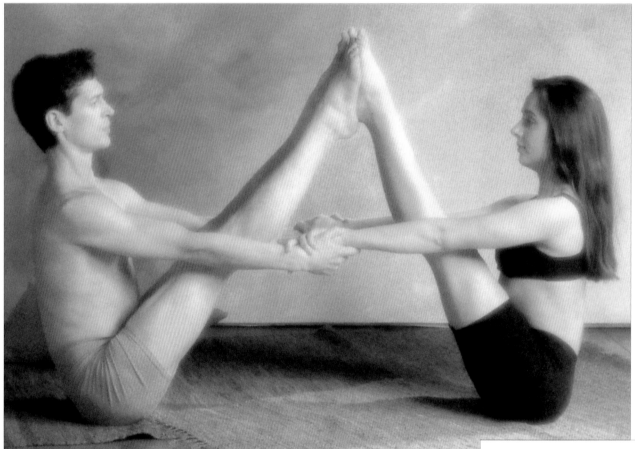

3. From this position proceed into the BOAT POSE. Lift your right foot and press the sole into your partner's left foot. Press, foot to foot, carefully maintaining your balance and straighten your leg up inside your arms, with a strong stretch in the arms.

4. Repeat with your left foot and leg (and your partner's right foot and leg), while keeping the right (left) leg extended. Make sure both legs are together and hold for four to five breaths.

BOAT POSE

(*Sanskrit*: Navāsana)

THIS POSTURE LOOSELY RESEMBLES THAT OF A BOAT WITH OARS, HENCE ITS NAME.

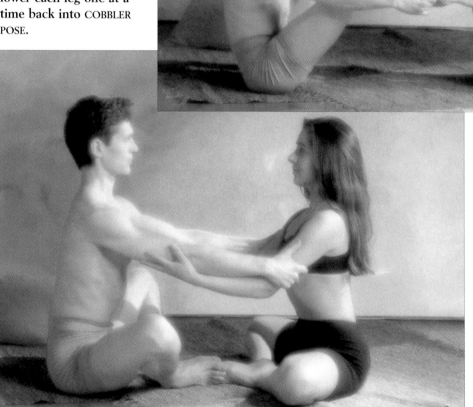

5. (right and below) Widen your legs apart, pressing your knees against your arms and hold for four to five breaths. Then bring the legs back together and lower each leg one at a time back into COBBLER POSE.

HELPFUL HINTS

• BEFORE YOU START this sequence, spend some time in COBBLER POSE just breathing gently together.

• TAKE YOUR TIME as you progress through the sequence. Balance is important, and the best way to achieve this is to keep the lower back in, shoulders back, arms well stretched and the gaze softly fixed.

• SYNCHRONIZE YOUR MOVEMENTS as you lift, and straighten one leg and then the other.

• SUPPORT AND GUIDE each other through the sequence.

6. As a counterstretch, one partner bends forward, stretching at the hips and resting their head on their partner's feet, if possible. The other partner leans over them, stretching out to hold their partner's hips. Relax into this pose and hold for four to five breaths.

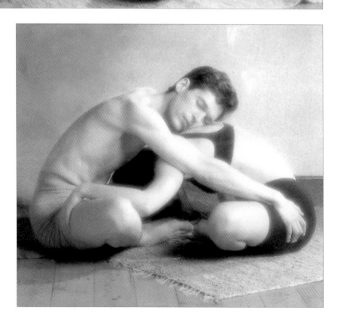

4. ENERGIZING

PHYSICAL EFFECTS

This sequence helps to develop flexibility in the body and improves stamina. It opens the chest and increases the capacity to breathe deeply. The shoulders and arms are stretched, and the pelvis is lifted. The postures are combined so that the male and female partners exchange roles: the man takes the passive role, helping to stabilize the woman in her strong WARRIOR POSE, offering gentle support and guidance. Then the roles reverse.

In the second part of the sequence the legs, hips and spine are stretched and relaxed.

The support of your partner in this strong sequence is essential as the forward bend can be greatly improved from a point of stability.

EMOTIONAL REFLECTIONS

By switching the action and support roles between the partners the exchange of male and female energy is developed and balanced. The sequence is vibrant and energizing, and encourages the development of overall strength and vitality.

MEDITATION
I am strong and invincible but need, and respect, my partner

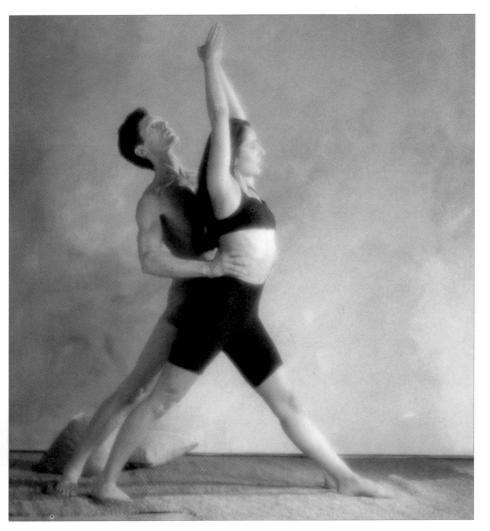

1. (left) Both partners stand, one behind the other, hips to hips, legs just over 3.5ft (1m) apart. Both turn to the left, rotating the right foot in with the left pointing forward. The hips and chest are in line with the left, outstretched foot. The front partner's arms are stretched up in line with the ears.

2. (opposite) Reach up and breathe. Both partners then bend their front legs, so that the thigh forms an angle of 90 degrees with the shin. The supporting partner assists by ensuring the front pelvis is lifted. Keep the back leg extended. A strong upward stretch is maintained throughout the body, with eyes, throat and jaw remaining soft. Breathe deeply for four to five breaths.

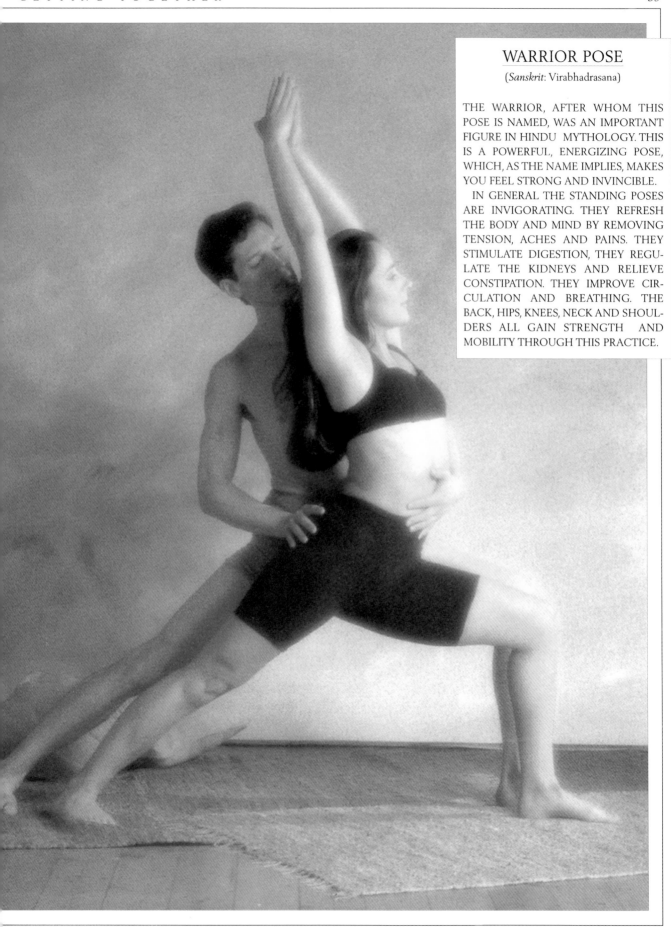

WARRIOR POSE
(*Sanskrit*: Virabhadrasana)

THE WARRIOR, AFTER WHOM THIS POSE IS NAMED, WAS AN IMPORTANT FIGURE IN HINDU MYTHOLOGY. THIS IS A POWERFUL, ENERGIZING POSE, WHICH, AS THE NAME IMPLIES, MAKES YOU FEEL STRONG AND INVINCIBLE.

IN GENERAL THE STANDING POSES ARE INVIGORATING. THEY REFRESH THE BODY AND MIND BY REMOVING TENSION, ACHES AND PAINS. THEY STIMULATE DIGESTION, THEY REGULATE THE KIDNEYS AND RELIEVE CONSTIPATION. THEY IMPROVE CIRCULATION AND BREATHING. THE BACK, HIPS, KNEES, NECK AND SHOULDERS ALL GAIN STRENGTH AND MOBILITY THROUGH THIS PRACTICE.

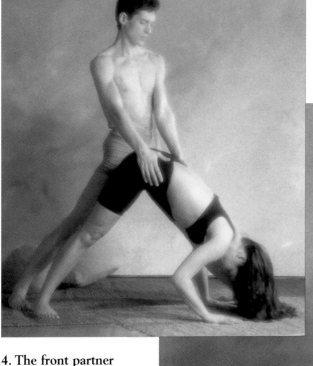

3. Both partners draw their left hips back, as the left leg is straightened. The front partner then stretches forward and down over the left leg, fully extends the trunk and takes the hands to the floor. The back partner supports the hips. Hold for four to five breaths.

4. The front partner then bends the front leg, places both hands one on top of the other on the bent leg thigh and gently pushes up to the upright position. Hold for a breath or two and then return to the first position.

5. Repeat with the right leg in front, then change with the supporting partner now performing the active role.

HELPFUL HINTS

• KEEP THE FEET really firm in this strong sequence. It is important always to move from a stable base, particularly when the upward stretch is so strong.

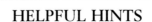

• IN THE FIRST part of the movement, when you stretch up in the WARRIOR POSE, it is important to ensure the tailbone remains tucked in so that the lower back doesn't strain. The pelvis has to lift up.

• KEEP THE BREATH constant throughout. It is easy to take short breaths into the upper chest in these strong poses, so think deep and low.

• HOLD THE POSE for the recommended number of breaths, but if you feel that you can benefit from staying longer, do so; if you experience too much strain come out sooner.

5. COMING TOGETHER

PHYSICAL EFFECTS

This is a good posture to do with a partner. Your combined support helps to achieve a full stretch and enables total relaxation. You need a strong base for the sequence; the outstretched leg should be firmly pressed into the floor.

This posture is toning for the liver, kidneys and spleen and aids digestion. The pelvis is opened, and the spine is extended.

This FORWARD BEND POSE is very calming and helps to remove fatigue by refreshing the brain.

Take the time to perform these movements slowly and with deep breaths.

EMOTIONAL REFLECTIONS

This sequence initially develops the feeling of being secure in your own space, yet together with your partner. In the final movement both partners acknowledge each other's comfort, care and support. The pose asserts each partner's separate identity within the awareness of their togetherness.

MEDITATION
I am apart and yet a part of you

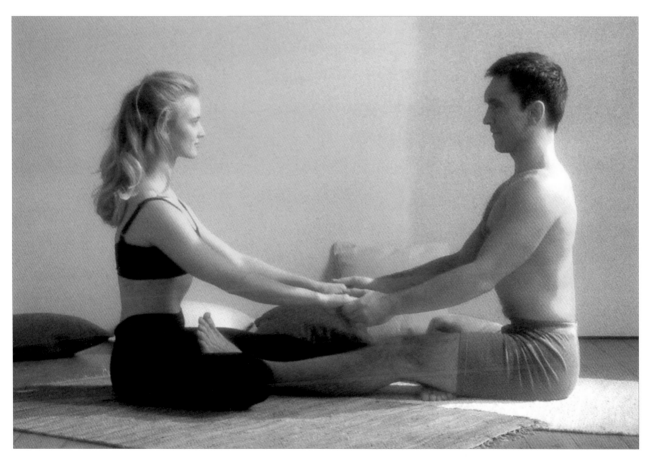

1. Sit on the floor, facing your partner. Extend the left leg and bend the right leg, placing the right heel in the groin.

Place the straight-leg heel against the other partner's bent-leg foot. Hold your partner's hands, keeping the arms

loosely relaxed. Stretch up and breathe deeply, keeping the spine straight and shoulders back.

2. Each partner lifts through the spine and turns towards their own bent leg. One hand is placed on the floor beyond the base of the spine; the other hand presses into the partner's outer knee to aid the lift and to keep stable in the pose. Hold for four to five breaths.

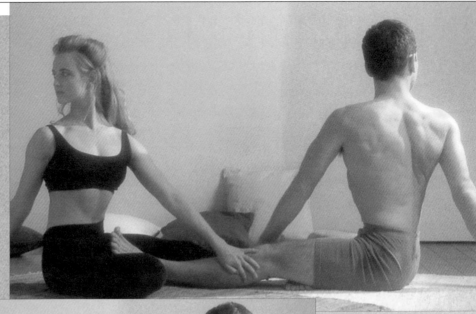

3. Each partner lifts and rotates the trunk in the opposite direction so they are looking beyond the straight-leg hip, with, again, one hand reaching behind and the other on their own straight-leg knee. Hold for four to five breaths.

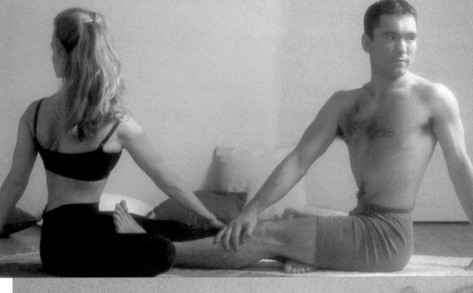

HELPFUL HINTS

• USE THE SUPPORT of a cushion or folded blanket under the buttocks if the lower back feels stiff.

• USE SOME SUPPORTIVE padding under the bended knee if it doesn't reach the floor.

• PLACE A FOLDED blanket or cushions under the lower partner's chest in the FORWARD BEND if there is strain in the lower back.

• BREATHE SOFTLY AND quietly in the FORWARD BEND, gradually allowing your body to release more and more.

• TRY TO KEEP the straight leg extended throughout the pose, but if at first this is too difficult, bend it slightly.

4.(below) Return to the first position and lean into a FORWARD BEND, keeping the straight leg well extended, lifting the spine and the chest and taking the buttock bones back. One partner stretches over the other. Hold for as long as is comfortable.

5. Return to the first position, reverse legs and repeat the sequence.

The internal organs

There are a great many similarities between the ancient Hindu and Chinese traditions, none more apparent than in their approaches to the nature of energy (in yoga: 'prana', in Chinese medicine: 'qi') and function of the internal organs.

In both traditions, qi, or prana, is our vital life force, which circulates through meridians, invisible channels in the body through which qi flows to the organs, adjusting and harmonizing their activity. If the qi is moving normally through the body, our bodies are protected against illness. Blockages in the flow of qi lead to disease.

Each organ has physical and emotional qualities. The heart, for instance, is not only the major organ in the circulatory system but also the center of our emotions. Blockages can lead to excessive mood swings and outbursts as well as physical problems such as angina or artery disease.

Lung problems can manifest themselves physically as colds, influenza and asthma, or emotionally as an overwhelming sense of sadness. The liver and gall bladder are linked, and ailments associated with them include gastric ulcers, eye conditions and stomach ache. Emotionally the liver and gall bladder are associated with depression, anger and frustration.

Kidney disorders are expressed emotionally in fear and anxiety, and physically with ear problems and infertility. The spleen and stomach are connected to anxiety, pensiveness and stress, and disfunction often manifests itself in the body through general weakness, lassitude, diarrhea and anemia.

Yoga asanas, and the sequences we have developed here, stimulate the internal organs and meridians through twists and stretches, clearing any potential or actual blockages to promote a balance of energies and optimum health.

FORWARD BEND

(*Sanskrit*: Janu Sirsasana)

'JANU' MEANS 'KNEE' AND 'SIRSA' IS 'HEAD', AND THE FORWARD BEND INVOLVES BRINGING THE HEAD TO THE KNEE. THIS SEQUENCE IS PARTICULARLY BENEFICIAL IF YOU ARE FEELING RUN DOWN OR SLIGHTLY LETHARGIC.

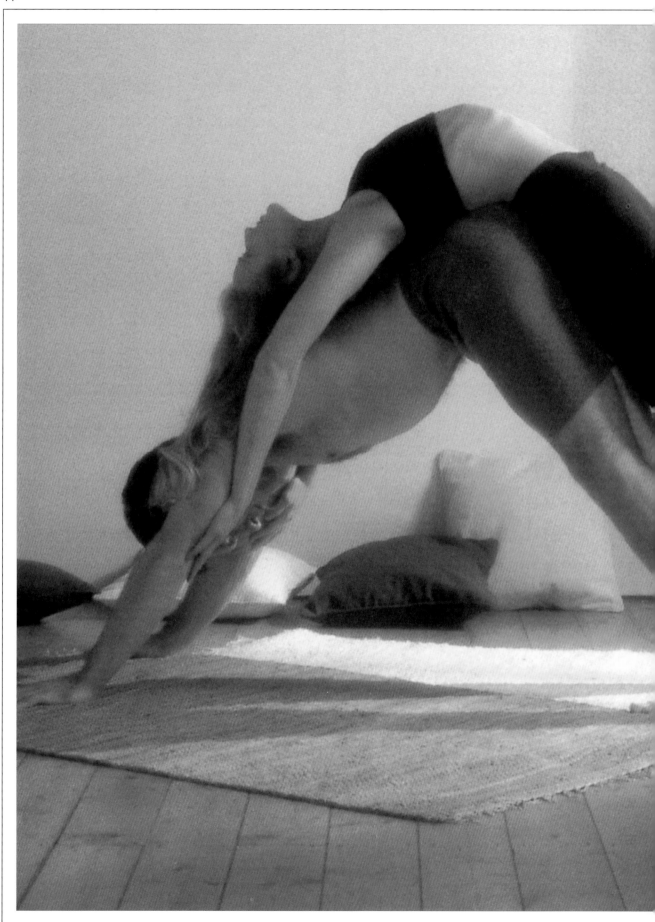

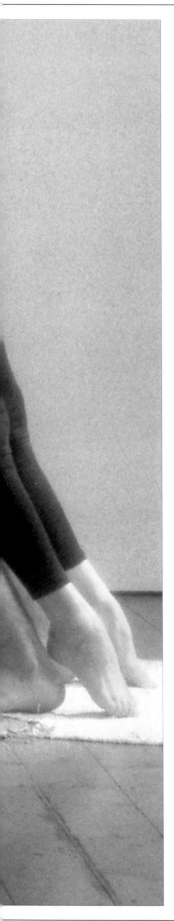

STARTING THE DAY TOGETHER

THE STATE OF BEING awake is one in which we are sensitive to ourselves and to those around us. This sensitivity and awareness is one of the main conditions of loving. Unfortunately a vast number of people today are, emotionally speaking, half asleep when awake and half awake when asleep. To be fully active in thought and feeling is indispensable to the art of loving.

Words can be misunderstood.
Without speaking, without understanding,
lovers can find each other.

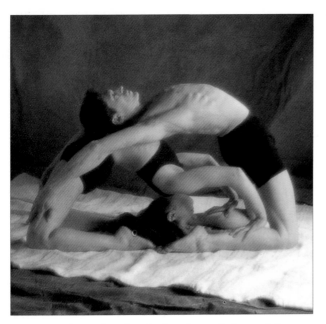

If we are alive, clear-headed and in a balanced frame of mind, we are open to the gift of love

1. RECEIVING

PHYSICAL EFFECTS

This pose presents the best possible way to start your day together. It is a simple upward stretch, using the breath and taking in as much oxygen as you can to recharge your body after a night's sleep. With the support of your partner's back to lift, stretch and release, you will feel revitalized and ready for the day ahead.

The upward stretch of the body will help to center your natural energies. As you reach up, you will expand your chest, which will help to increase your capacity to breathe deeply. The spine and neck are stretched, as are the muscles of the shoulders and arms. The upward pull through the legs will firm the thighs and hips.

As you lower the arms and twist to one side, then the other, the abdominal organs are gently toned and stretched too.

EMOTIONAL REFLECTIONS

In this sequence you are opening your body and mind to the day. It has a centering and focusing effect, overcoming the heaviness of the night and filling the body with renewed vigor.

MEDITATION
I am ready to receive the day

HELPED HINTS

Consequently, in any loving relationship, early mornings are extremely important. If we are not awake, totally, to each other, mornings can be a minefield of tensions and loose emotions. Minor conflicts are avoided because time is short. Both physically and emotionally we are at our lowest ebb, cluttered by the toxins and mental cobwebs of the previous night. Meaningful communication is often non-existent, and seemingly small problems can, and often do, carry over, day by day, gathering intensity until they erupt in anger.

At this most difficult time, the benefits are huge if we can manage to practice *The Art of Sensual Yoga*. The sequences are balancing and invigorating, and help to clear our bodies and minds for the day ahead. The emphasis is on balance, support and communication. As we saw in chapter 3, 'Getting Together', where verbal communication between partners is difficult or strained, the physical contact provides a bridge.

The exercises ease tension and anger out of the parts of the body that store them, areas such as the neck, shoulders and hips. They center the emotions and focus the mind for the day. The movements are positively energizing; a perfect way to start the day. If we are alive, clear-headed and in a balanced frame of mind, we are open to the gift of love.

• TAKE YOUR TIME with this first stretch of the day. Breathe quietly together for a while, slowly synchronizing your breath. Be aware of each other.

• AS YOU REACH up, allow your bodies gently to stretch together. Remember to draw your abdomen in and up as you raise your arms.

• AS YOU TWIST to the side, maintain firm contact with your hips and your outstretched arms.

• AS WITH ALL sequences, keep your eyes, throat and jaw soft, your breath regular and deep.

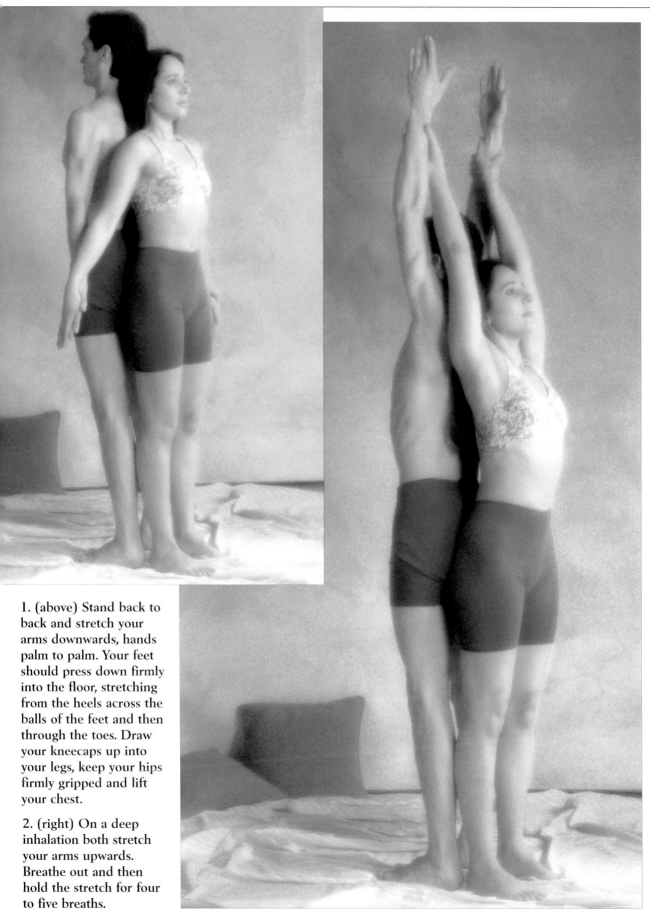

1. (above) Stand back to
back and stretch your
arms downwards, hands
palm to palm. Your feet
should press down firmly
into the floor, stretching
from the heels across the
balls of the feet and then
through the toes. Draw
your kneecaps up into
your legs, keep your hips
firmly gripped and lift
your chest.

2. (right) On a deep
inhalation both stretch
your arms upwards.
Breathe out and then
hold the stretch for four
to five breaths.

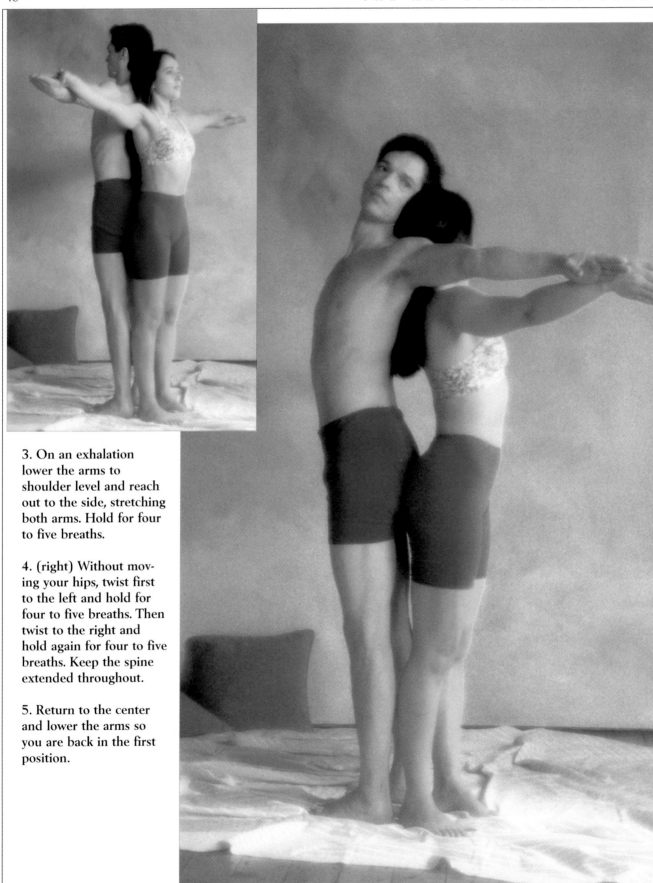

3. On an exhalation lower the arms to shoulder level and reach out to the side, stretching both arms. Hold for four to five breaths.

4. (right) Without moving your hips, twist first to the left and hold for four to five breaths. Then twist to the right and hold again for four to five breaths. Keep the spine extended throughout.

5. Return to the center and lower the arms so you are back in the first position.

2. REACHING

PHYSICAL EFFECTS

This is a development from sequence one, in which the stretch through the legs and hips is increased. You are now facing each other, and this pose calls for more mutual support.

This sequence will help to relieve stiffness in the legs and hip joints as the trunk bends forward.

The spine is extended, and the support of your partner will help you to release and extend further. In this sequence you are dependent on each other for firm support and stability.

The second part of the sequence, in which one leg is taken in front of the other, provides an excellent stretch for the hamstring muscles in the backs of the legs.

EMOTIONAL REFLECTIONS

The sequence develops from a stable standing position, in which each partner feels strong and secure in themselves. By reaching out they give their trust to each other in a mutual embrace.

MEDITATION
I reach out and embrace the day

1. Stand facing each other. Place your hands on your partner's shoulders; your partner should put their hands on your hips.

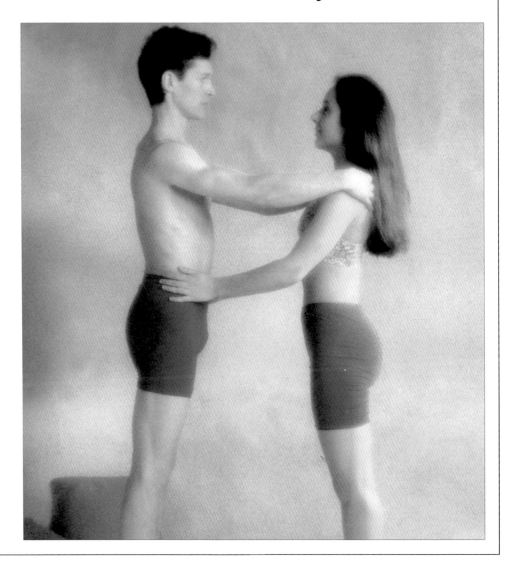

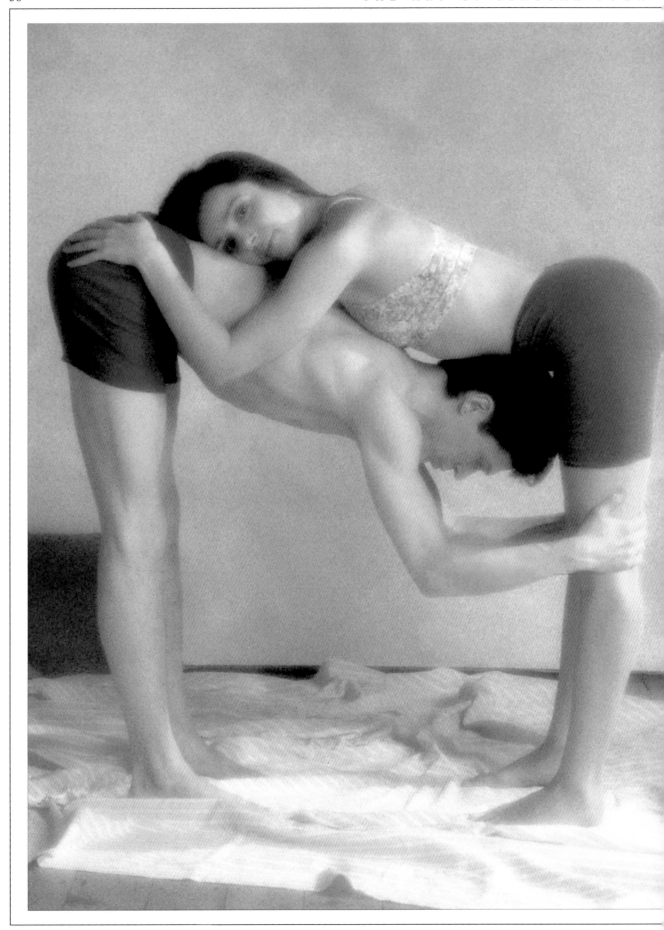

2. (opposite) Bend forward to a horizontal position, holding the back of your partner's thighs. Your partner then bends forward to lie across your extended trunk, holding your hips and stretching along your back. Hold for four or five breaths.

3. Slowly come back to the first position. Bend forward again so that your partner lies on top this time. Hold for four or five breaths.

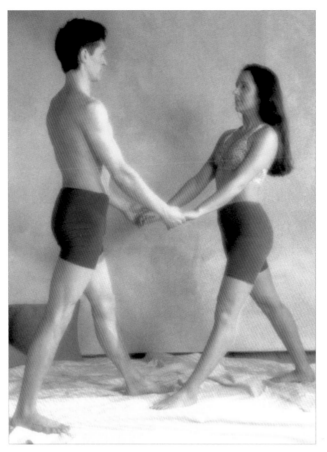

4. Come back up to the first position and hold your partner's hands. Each of you takes the left leg forward, while keeping your right leg extended back, with the right foot turned in to an angle of 45 degrees. Your hips and chest should face towards each other.

5. (below) Bend forward and extend towards each other; as before, one partner stretching over the other. Hold the position for four to five breaths.

6. Lift up and repeat sequences 4 and 5 with your right leg in front.

HELPFUL HINTS

• MAINTAIN A STRONG upward stretch through the legs. If there is any strain in the backs of the legs, feel free to bend them from time to time.

• KEEP BREATHING STEADILY throughout the pose and give each other total support.

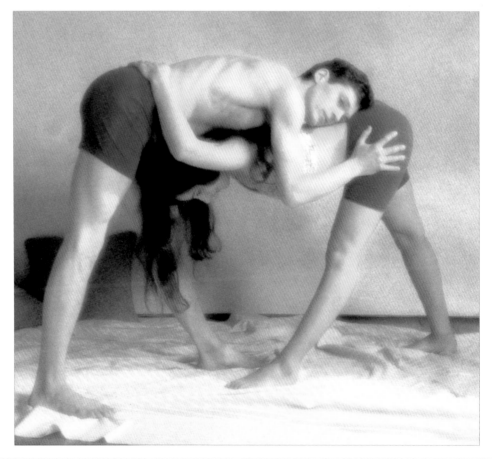

3. CHANGE

PHYSICAL EFFECTS

This sequence of movements is wonderful for toning the lower back.

It reduces flab around the abdominal area and tones the abdominal muscles, helping to relieve gastric problems.

There is an excellent stretch for the legs, arms and chest.

This is a clearing and energizing sequence of movements.

EMOTIONAL REFLECTIONS

Toning the stomach develops our ability to accept change and to receive the new. Strengthening the stomach improves our capacity to assimilate new facts, new events and new emotions.

MEDITATION
I am ready for change

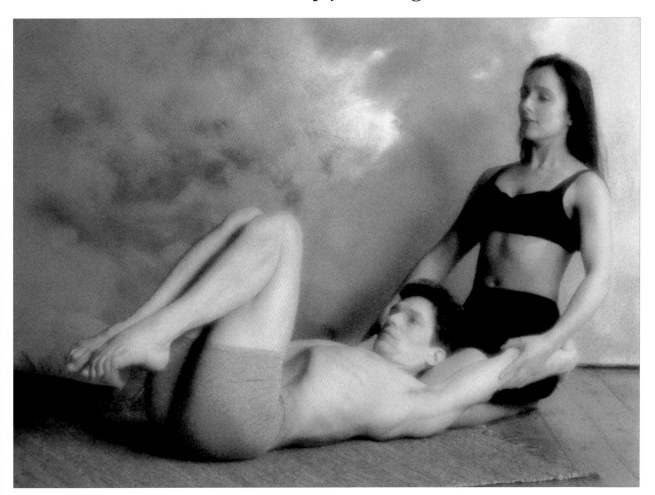

1. Lie flat on your back on the floor and stretch your arms back, holding your partner's waist. Bend your knees to your chest. The supportive partner sits on their heels; taking care not to strain, they use their body gently to stretch the reclining partner's upper arms.

2. Push your waist into the floor and take your legs to a vertical position. Your partner should help keep a strenuous stretch through your ribs and spine by strongly drawing your upper arms back. Take four to five breaths in this position.

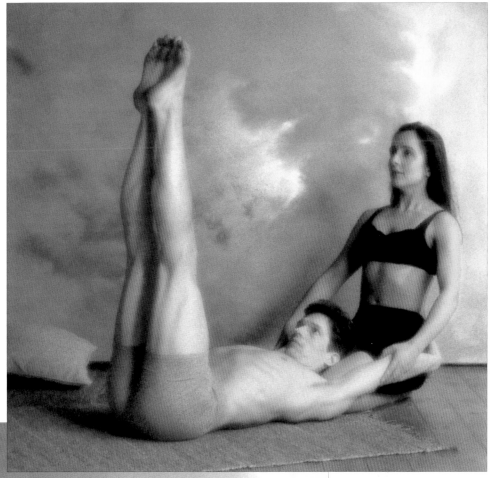

3. Take a deep breath in, and on the exhalation lower your legs to a 60-degree angle and hold them in this position for two breaths. Remember to stretch strongly into your feet and keep your waist pressing down towards the floor.

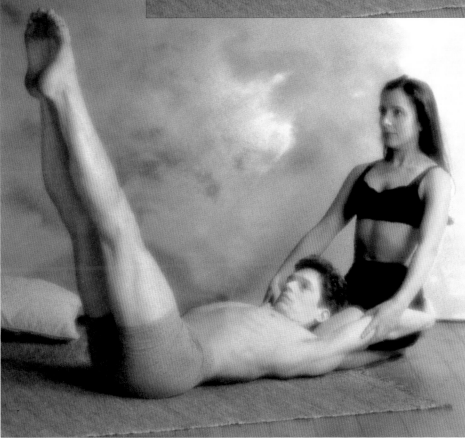

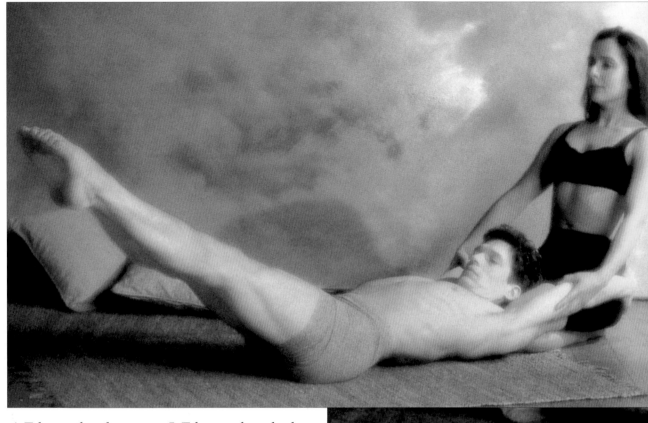

4. Take another deep breath, and on the exhalation take your legs down to an angle of 30 degrees. Hold for two breaths, keeping a strong stretch in the legs and trunk.

5. Take your legs slowly down to the floor. Your partner should continue to stretch your arms back.

6. Bend your legs to your chest and draw your shins to your thighs. Your partner should come round to the front and press down on to your shins to relieve any strain in the lower back.

7. Switch roles.

HELPFUL HINTS

• IF YOU EXPERIENCE any backache during this sequence, see if you can release it by pushing your lower back into the floor more firmly. If this doesn't work, try doing the sequence with your knees slightly bent. If there is still discomfort, do not continue.

• AT ALL TIMES keep the throat, jaw and eyes soft. There is a strong inclination to grip in the throat and jaw with this sequence so you need to consciously relax in this area so there is no strain in the head, neck and shoulders.

• KEEP THE BREATH steady throughout.

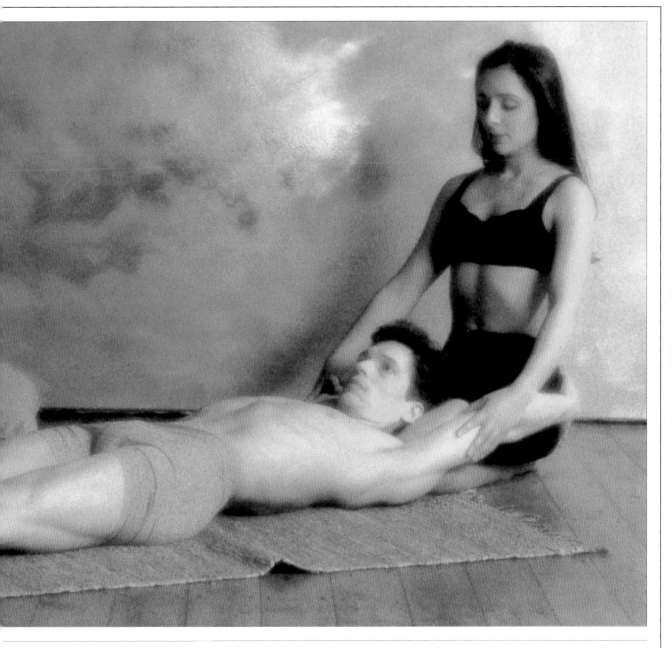

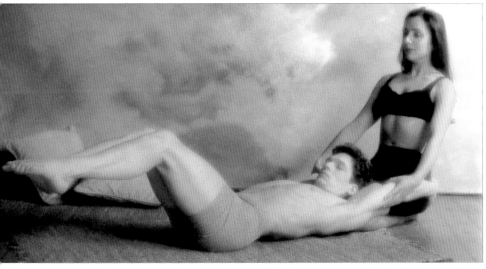

4. LIFE FORCE

PHYSICAL EFFECTS

It is recommended that you warm up with the previous sequences before commencing here. You will need the stability and openness achieved in the earlier stages to appreciate this one fully and be comfortable in it.

This is an invigorating sequence that will help give you strength and flexibility in your body. The extension of the spine is strong, the legs are stretched to the maximum, and the internal organs are toned.

Your partner's support will help you to extend fully from a stable position.

EMOTIONAL REFLECTIONS

In yoga philosophy life force is stored in the base of the spine. This energy is called *Kundalini* (Sanskrit: 'the coiled one'). Blockages in the spine inhibit this vital force, leading to lethargy and a loss of joy in life. The spine extensions in this sequence release the blockages and help free your life force.

MEDITATION
I am filled with the energy of the universe

1. Stand one behind the other, feet just about 3–3.5ft (1m) wide, hips to hips, shoulders to chest.

2. Both turn the right foot slightly in and the left leg completely out to the side. Your left heel should be in line with your right middle instep. The active partner raises their arms out to the side and stretches through them to the tips of the fingers, while keeping the wrists level with the shoulders. The supporting partner keeps their hands on your hips, offering stability and balance.

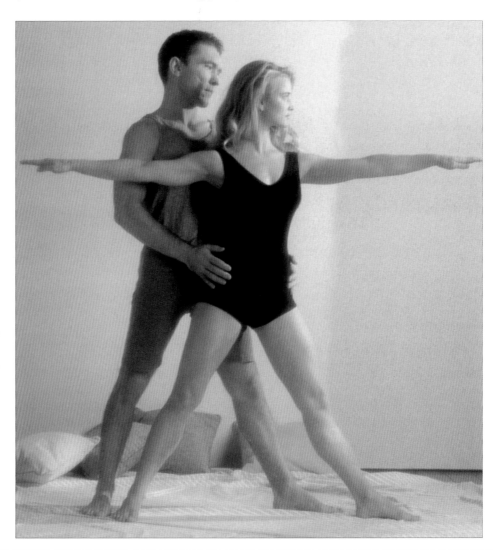

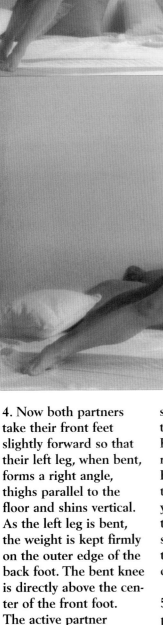

3. The supporting partner places their left hand on your right shoulder as you slowly take your body down to the left side, in line with your front leg. Place your left hand round your ankle and your right around your supporting partner's shoulders, using your ankle and partner for support. Hold for four to five breaths.

HELPFUL HINTS

• IN THIS SEQUENCE your supporting partner should help to keep the back and hips in line, so that the tailbone aligns with the back of the head.

• GIVE EACH OTHER firm support in this sequence as it is strong. Breathe and extend together as you go into the pose.

• KEEP A VERY firm grounding action in your feet, so you have a stable base from which to extend.

• AS YOU MOVE into the final part of the sequence think of a straight line all the way from your back heel through to the back of your head and stretch along it.

• KEEP THE SHOULDER-BLADES tucked in and the shoulders turned back throughout the sequence, so the chest remains open.

• YOUR EYES, THROAT and jaw should remain soft and the breath steady.

• HOLD THE POSE only as long as is reasonably comfortable.

4. Now both partners take their front feet slightly forward so that their left leg, when bent, forms a right angle, thighs parallel to the floor and shins vertical. As the left leg is bent, the weight is kept firmly on the outer edge of the back foot. The bent knee is directly above the center of the front foot. The active partner stretches their trunk towards their bent knee. Keep both sides of the rib-cage extended evenly. Reach your left hand to the floor. (Initially balance yourself with your fingertips, but with practice you should eventually be able to place the whole palm on the floor.)

5. Find balance and support with the help of your partner, and hold the pose for four to five breaths.

6. Inhale as you come out by pushing into the front foot and then gracefully perform the pose on the other side, keeping a continuity of movement.

7. Now reverse roles.

5. NOURISHMENT

PHYSICAL EFFECTS

This sequence benefits both partners as the combination provides a strong stretch in its second section.

In the DOG POSE the ankles and legs are well stretched, thus removing stiffness in these areas.

The shoulders are strongly stretched and the abdominal muscles toned and firmed.

This sequence nourishes the brain cells and eases fatigue.

Halfway through roles reverse, and the supporting partner becomes the supported one. When the now supported partner stretches their back along their partner's spine, this helps to open the diaphragm and then, in the later part of the sequence, fully opens the upper chest. There is benefit, too, in the support received from the prone partner.

This is a rejuvenating series of movements.

EMOTIONAL REFLECTIONS

The supporting partner in this sequence is fixed and solid in both DOG POSE and CHILD'S POSE. Imagine a tree, rooted in the ground, drawing its energy from the earth and providing nourishment, shelter and support.

MEDITATION
I am strong and ready to give

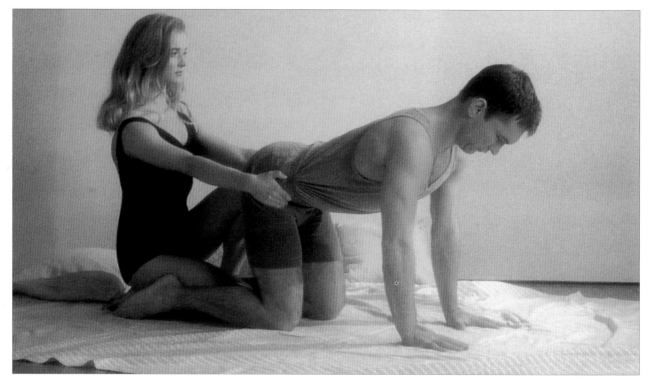

1. Position yourself on your hands and knees and extend your spine. Your partner sits behind you, in whatever position is comfortable, and takes hold of your hips and stretches them back. Hold for four to five breaths.

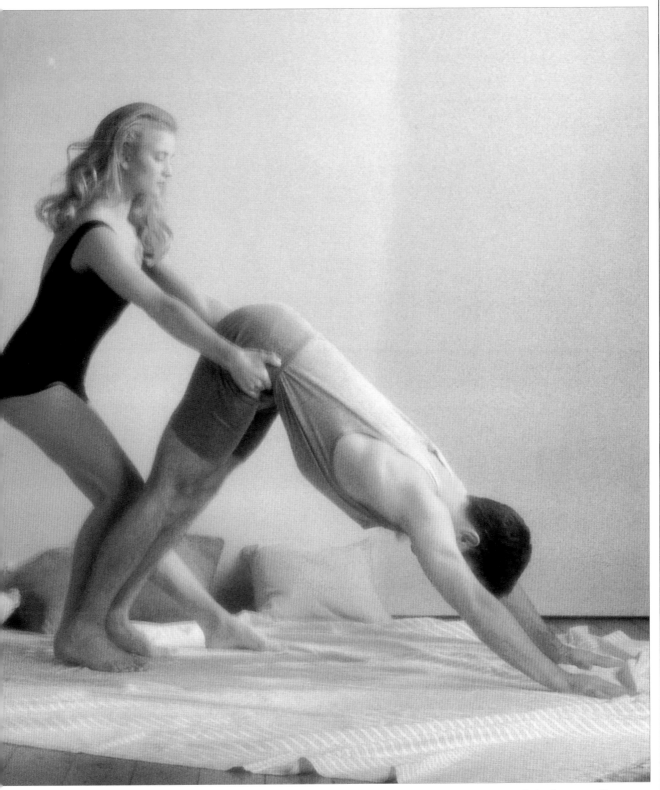

2. Your partner stands up and in doing so draws your hips upwards into the DOG POSE so the legs are straight. Press your heels and hands into the floor, while lifting the back ribs up towards the hips and away from the shoulders. Move your chest back towards legs. The trunk now forms a V shape, with the legs stretching away from the extended heels and the trunk lifting up and away from the hands.

Keeping the hips lifted with the help of your partner, stretch the shins and thighs away from the trunk.

Relax the head and neck. Breathe steadily and hold for four to five breaths.

DOG POSE

(Sanskrit: Adho Mukha Svanasana)

'ADHO MUKHA' MEANS 'HAVING THE FACE DOWNWARD'; 'SVAN' MEANS 'DOG'. THE POSE RESEMBLES A DOG STRETCHING ITSELF WITH ITS HEAD AND FORELEGS DOWN, POINTED FORWARD, AND ITS BACK LEGS STANDING ON THE GROUND – HENCE THE NAME. THIS CLASSIC POSE CALMS THE HEART AND REJUVENATES THE BODY, WHILE THE INCREASED BLOOD FLOW NOURISHES THE BRAIN.

3. (right and far right) Your partner goes around to the front of you and places their feet between your hands, resting their hips gently on your upper spine. They then lie along your spine, taking their head back over your hips, while stretching out their legs. Hold for four to five breaths.

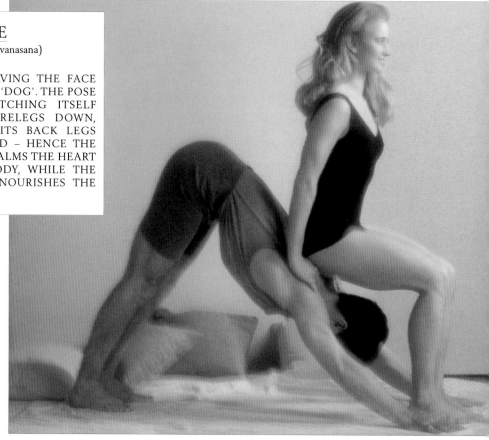

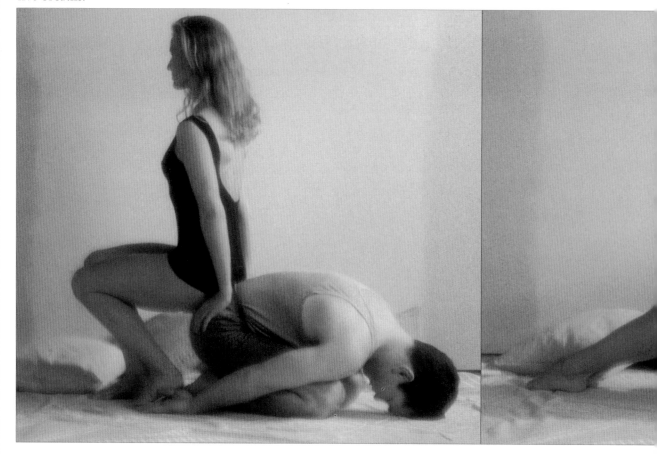

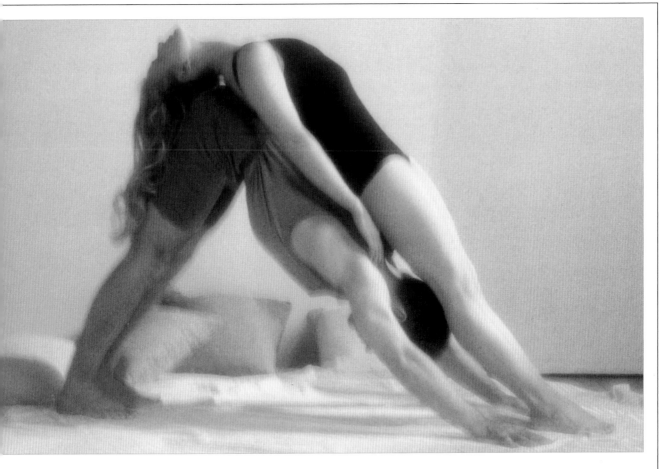

4. (far left and left) Move into CHILD'S POSE. Your partner sits on your hips and stretches their trunk over your spine with arms and legs outstreached. Hold for four to five breaths.

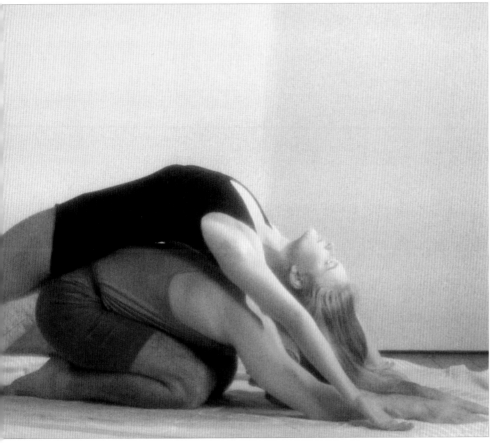

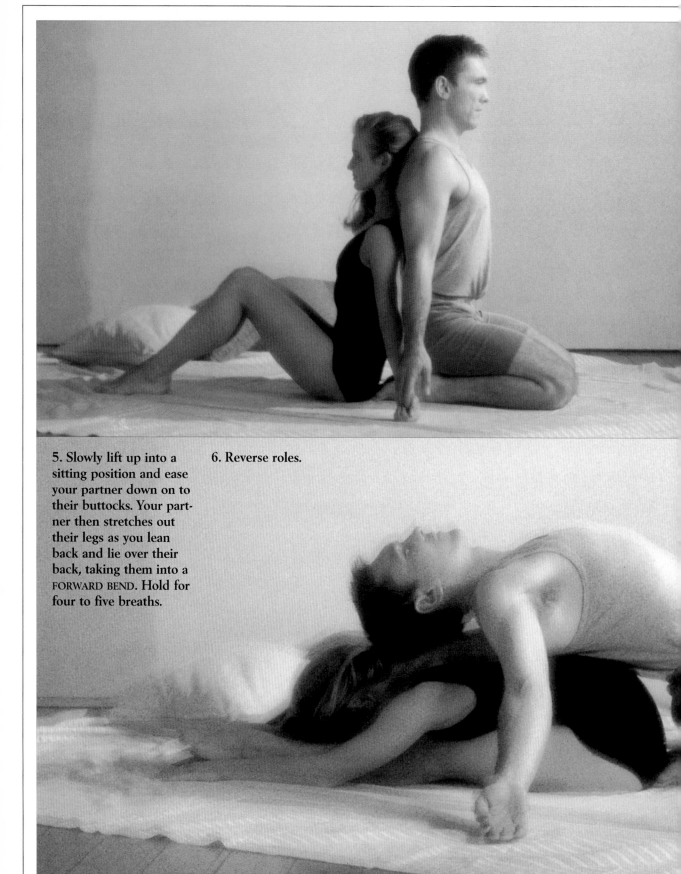

**5. Slowly lift up into a
sitting position and ease
your partner down on to
their buttocks. Your partner then stretches out
their legs as you lean
back and lie over their
back, taking them into a
FORWARD BEND. Hold for
four to five breaths.**

6. Reverse roles.

HELPFUL HINTS

• REMEMBER TO MAINTAIN a strong, upward stretch in this pose, while keeping the breath steady and soft throughout.

• IN THE DOG pose draw the abdominal muscles back towards the spine and the diaphragm up towards the chest.

• TRY TO KEEP the head and neck passive throughout the various stages of the pose, with the eyes, throat and jaw soft.

• BE SENSITIVE TO each other's needs throughout the sequence, giving just enough support and weight.

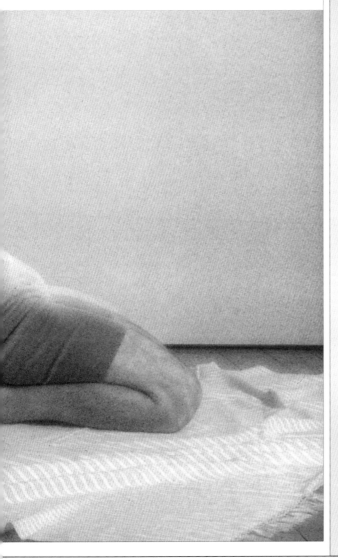

The spine

Back pain is endemic in western society. More time and resources are taken up with the treatment of it than with almost any other ailment. Spinal problems are familiar to many of us and include sciatica, slipped disc, migraine, lumbago, neck ache and stiffness in the upper shoulders. An awareness of the spine and its functions is essential to well-being.

The spine is the central supporting system of the body – the scaffold that holds the body upright and protects the organs. It contains 34 vertebrae, which form an S-shaped curve, all linked by powerful muscles and ligaments. These give the back support, strength and flexibility and are vital for the protection of the spinal cord. Between each of the vertebra there is a little cushion, shaped like a squashed golfball, called an inter-vertebral disc. Its task is to absorb shock and to prevent the bones from grinding against each other. A healthy spine involves strong muscles, good posture, flexible joints and freedom from stress and tension.

The leg raises in the CHANGE sequence (page 52) will strengthen the back muscles and improve spinal support. The triangular pose in LIFE FORCE (page 56) improves sideways flexibility and stretches all the lateral ligaments and muscles. The adapted DOG POSE in NOURISHMENT (page 58) stretches the entire spine and back muscles and relieves inter-vertebral compression. The CHILD'S POSE (page 24) is a good all-round back stretch, which can relieve strain in the lumbar region, and the CORPSE POSE (page 71) removes all stress from the spine and restores its natural symmetry.

Most of the yoga sequences in this book have the effect of strengthening the spine, improving flexibility and stretching and releasing the back muscles. A strong back and correct posture promotes good health and a positive approach towards a stress-free life.

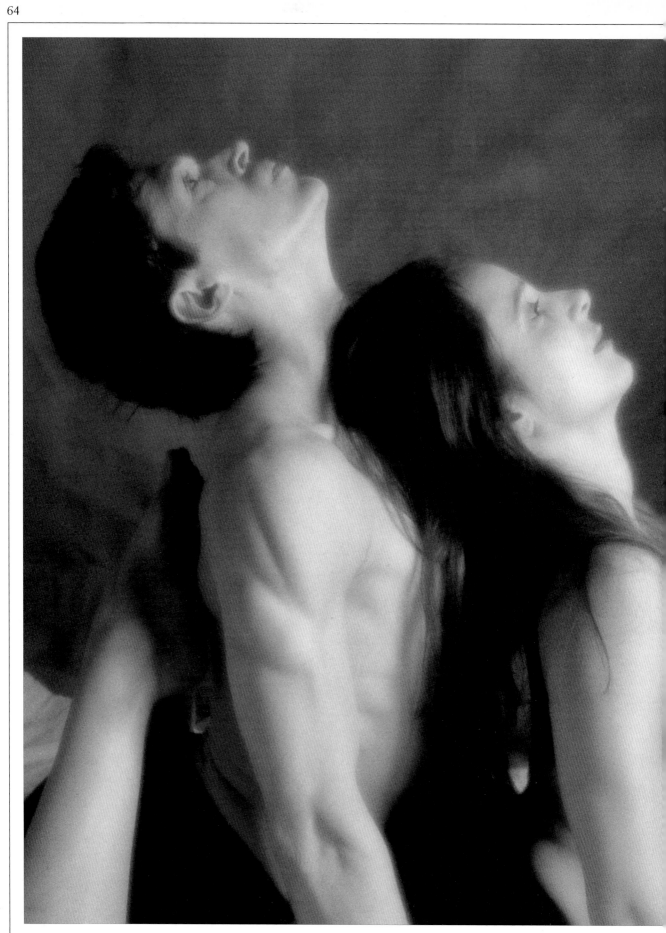

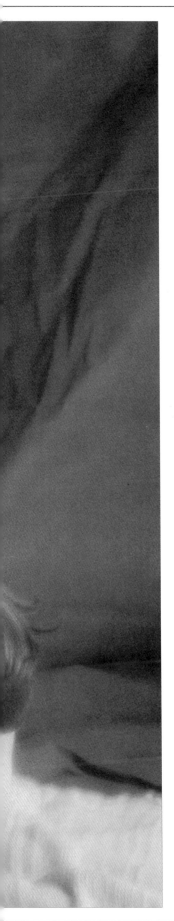

THE BREATH OF LIFE

Breath is life. We can live for days without food or water, but deprive us of breath for a matter of minutes, and we die. It is astonishing how little attention we pay in day-to-day existence to the importance of breathing correctly. The main function of the breath is to bring more oxygen to the blood and to provide vital energy. Through the practice of the art of breath control we have developed a series of exercises especially intended to meet these needs and keep the body healthy.

Receiving is a kind of giving.
Give as if receiving and receive as if giving.

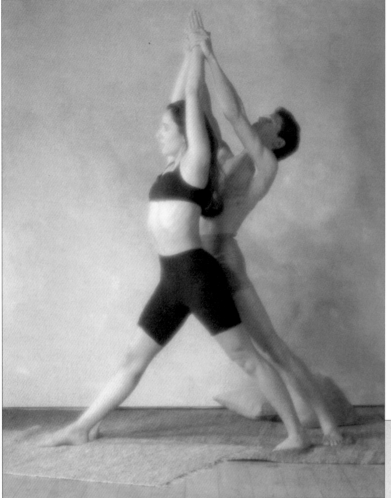

brings into play the whole of our lungs. When we exhale, the abdomen contracts and the diaphragm moves up, massaging the heart; when we inhale, the abdomen expands and the diaphragm moves down, massaging the abdominal organs.

Breathing exercises teach us how to control the mind. When we are angry or scared, our breathing is shallow, rapid and irregular; conversely, when we are relaxed, or deep in thought, our breathing becomes slow. This is easy to test yourselves. Listen for a moment to the lowest sound in the room. It becomes clear that, in concentrating, we unconsciously slow down, or even suspend, our breathing.

Since our state of mind is reflected in the way we breathe, it follows that by controlling the breath we can

Breath is life, and through breath control we can revitalize our bodies, steady our emotions and clarify our minds

There are three basic types of breathing: clavicular (shallow), intercostal (middle) and abdominal (deep). A full breath combines all three, beginning with a deep breath and continuing the inhalation through the intercostal and clavicular areas. Most of us have forgotten how to breathe properly. We inhale shallowly, through the mouth, and make little or no use of the diaphragm – either lifting the shoulders or contracting the abdomen. In this way just a small amount of oxygen is taken in, and only the top of the lungs is used.

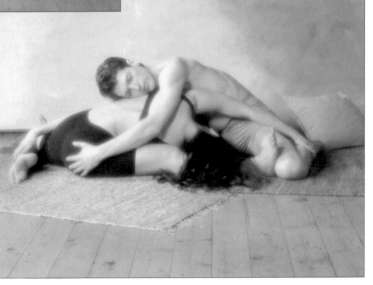

Breathing correctly means breathing through the nose and keeping the mouth closed. It involves a full inhalation and exhalation that learn to improve our mental resilience. By regulating our breathing we thus not only increase our intake of oxygen but also prepare ourselves for the practice of concentration and meditation. Breathing revitalizes the body, steadies the emotions and clarifies the mind.

1. SITTING BREATHING

PHYSICAL EFFECTS

If time is short this simple sequence will work to instill a quiet sense of calm in both of you. It will help to revitalize your whole system. If you have time to spare, then, as a more leisurely alternative, go on to the next sequence, Lying Breathing.

In Sitting Breathing your spine is stretched, and any stiffness in the back is eased. Your chest is gently opened. Try to make the duration of your inhalation and exhalation equal in length.

EMOTIONAL REFLECTIONS

This sequence is a gentle coming together for you as a couple. A tranquil time for both of you to pursue the elemental feeling of being alive, just by breathing together.

During the following breathing and relaxation sequences imagine that you are inhaling pure, white, cleansing light and exhaling all your negative emotions.

MEDITATION
I am filled with pure, clear energy

1. Sit back to back, spines lengthening into each other (backs of hands resting on knees) and shoulder to shoulder. The lower part of the spine should lift, and the lower abdomen should be drawn back. Lift the rib-cage, breast-bone and collar-bone. Bring the front armpits and the chest forward. Tuck the bottom of the shoulder-blades in and draw the shoulders back towards your partner's. Rest your heads one against the other. Keep the backs of your necks extended.

2. Watch the breath rise and fall and synchronize this with your partner. Breathe together softly and slowly and feel the expansion of your partner's back ribs as they move with the breath. Allow your eyes to sink down into their sockets as the eyelids close, taking the gaze inwards.

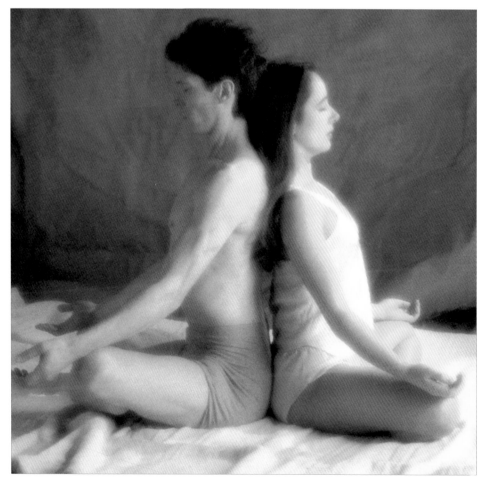

3. Focus all your attention on the simple rise and fall of the breath.

4. Sit breathing in this position for about a minute or two.

5. One partner takes the supporting role and sits behind the other, both with crossed legs.

6. Place your hands gently on your partner's diaphragm. The active partner should breathe into and across the palms of your hands and lean back gently into the supporting partner's body but keep the spine straight. Take four or five deep breaths in this position and then breathe normally for a few breaths.

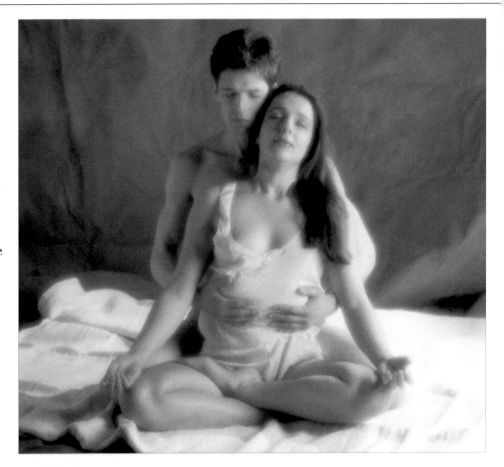

7. Place your hands lightly on your partner's side ribs. Breathe across the chest into the palms of the hands. Push them gently to the side with the breath. Take four or five deep breaths and then breathe normally.

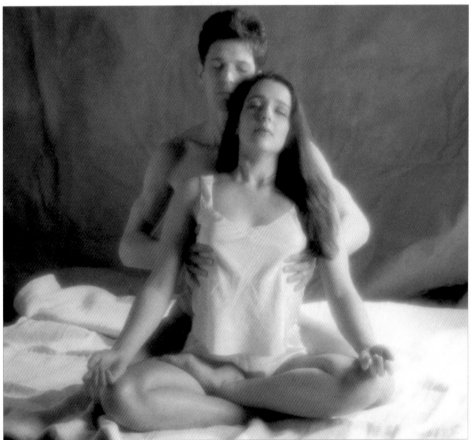

8. Place your hands lightly on your partner's top chest, the heels of your hands resting lightly in their front armpits, fingertips on their collar-bones. Breathe into the heels of the hands, then into the fingertips. Breathe deeply for four or five breaths, then breathe normally.

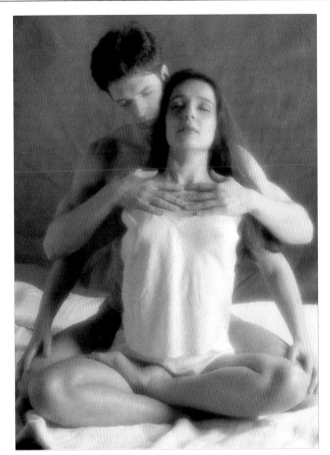

HELPFUL HINTS

• SIT ON A blanket if there is pressure on the lower back and add support under the knees if there is any strain on them.

• KEEP THE FOUNDATION of your pose firm by gently contracting the pelvic-floor muscles and sinking the buttock bones down into the floor. This helps to keep the tailbone lifted and thus the rest of the spine.

• BE SURE TO keep your throat, jaw, eyes and all the muscles of your face relaxed throughout the sequence.

9. Place one hand above your partner's navel and the other on their top chest. Breathe deeply, taking the breath from the lower to the upper hand. Take four or five deep breaths, then breathe normally. This completes the cycle.

10. Switch roles.

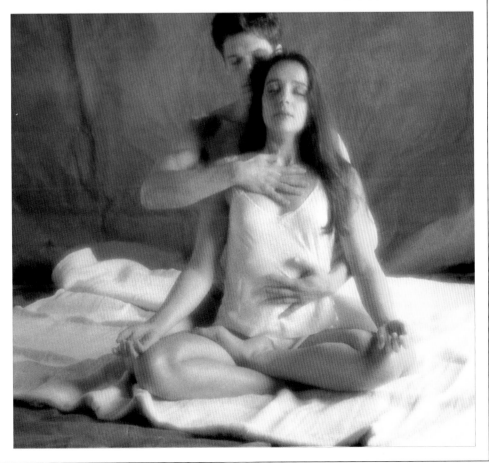

2. LYING BREATHING

PHYSICAL EFFECTS

With the opening of the chest and concentrated breathing the blood receives a greater supply of oxygen. One feels refreshed and revitalized. The nervous system is calmed and the mind stilled.

The abdominal organs are massaged as the abdomen expands and the diaphragm descends on inhalation. During exhalation the heart is massaged as the abdomen contracts and the diaphragm moves up.

EMOTIONAL REFLECTIONS

After completing this sequence you will become calm and at peace with yourself and partner. You will feel in control of your mind, all those busy thoughts stilled for a while.

MEDITATION
I am floating in a sea of calmness

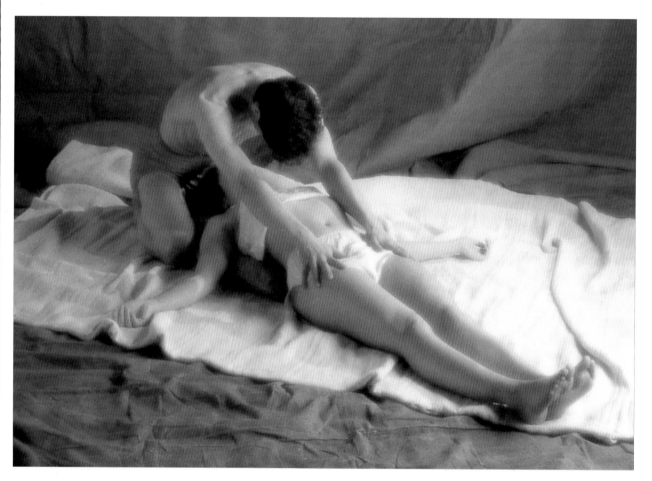

1. The reclining partner lies quietly in the CORPSE POSE before commencing the breathing exercises. The kneeling partner then gently presses the hip bones of the reclin-

ing partner down and away from them in order to extend the front of the body.

2. (opposite) Lay one hand on the abdomen, slightly above the navel. Breathe into this hand and, as you exhale, draw your abdomen back and up towards your chest.

Breathe slowly four to five times, then return to normal breathing.

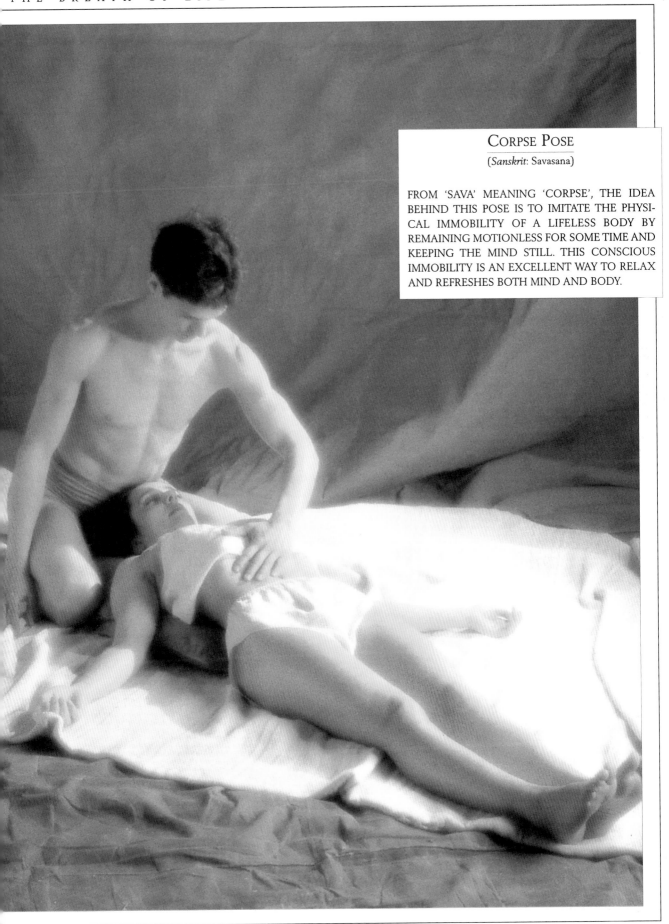

CORPSE POSE

(*Sanskrit*: Savasana)

FROM 'SAVA' MEANING 'CORPSE', THE IDEA BEHIND THIS POSE IS TO IMITATE THE PHYSICAL IMMOBILITY OF A LIFELESS BODY BY REMAINING MOTIONLESS FOR SOME TIME AND KEEPING THE MIND STILL. THIS CONSCIOUS IMMOBILITY IS AN EXCELLENT WAY TO RELAX AND REFRESHES BOTH MIND AND BODY.

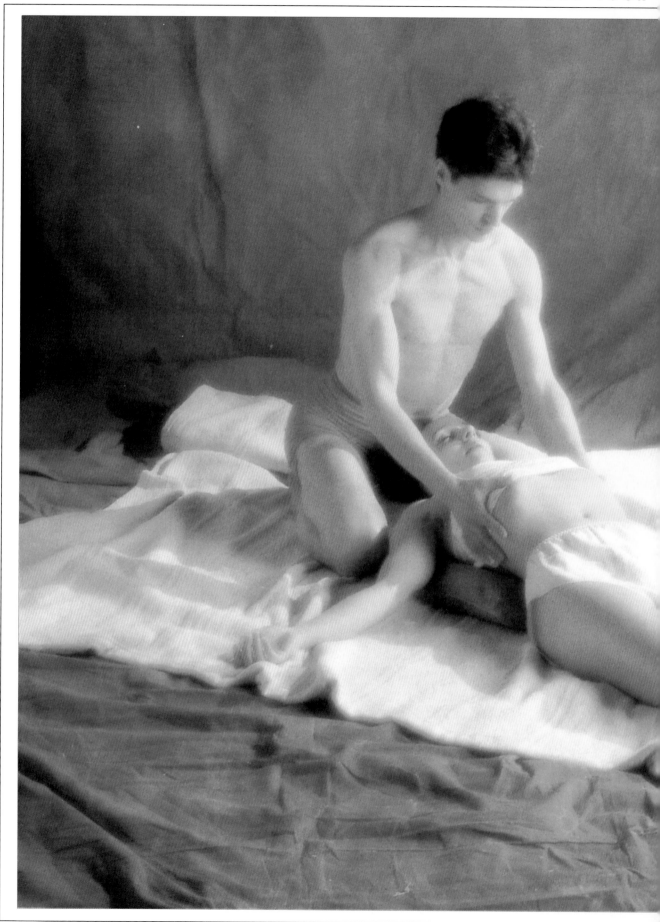

HELPFUL HINTS

• PREPARE SUPPORT FOR the reclining partner by folding a blanket lengthways or by using a couple of small cushions. The idea is to open the chest fully, so the padding needs to go under the back ribs and shoulders.

• EXHALE COMPLETELY BEFORE inhaling again. Allow the exhalation to be similar in length to the inhalation. Gently let the abdomen expand with the inhalation and draw in and up with the exhalation. Breathe only through the nose.

• KEEP THE BREATH smooth and even throughout each cycle.

• SEE IF YOU can be fully aware of how the whole body feels as you breathe. Consciously calm any restlessness or tension in your body with the breath. Keep softness and passivity in the eyes, throat, jaw and upper chest. Give yourself to your breath, the space around you and the support of your partner.

3. Lay both hands on your partner's side ribs. Breathe slowly into the hands taking the breath across the back ribs. Breathe slowly four or five times and then breathe normally.

4. Lay both hands on your partner's top chest, as in the sitting position. Breathe into the upper chest slowly four or five times and then return to normal breathing.

5. Take a long slow breath all the way from the navel to the collarbones, hold for five seconds and exhale slowly.

6. Roll over to your right side and rest in the fetal position for a short time.

7. Your partner removes their support so you are lying with your spine flat on the floor with your legs bent and feet on the floor. This eases the spine back in the usual position.

8. Switch roles when you are ready.

RELAXATION

Living with mind and body relaxed is our natural state, our birthright – it is only the pace of our lives that has made us forget. Those who retain the art possess the key to good health, vitality and peace of mind, because relaxation is a tonic for the whole being, liberating vast resources of energy.

The state of our minds and the condition of our bodies are intimately linked. If our muscles are relaxed, then our mind must be free of tension too. If the mind is anxious, then the body suffers too. All action originates in the mind. When the mind receives a stimulus that alerts it to the need for action, it sends a message via the nerves to contract the muscles in readiness. In the hustle and bustle of the modern world the mind is continuously bombarded with stimuli, which may cause us to freeze in the alerted 'fight or flight' pattern of response. As a result many people spend much of their lives – even when asleep – in a state of physical and mental tension.

Everyone has their own particular trouble spots, whether it is a clenched jaw, a furrowed brow, or a stiff neck. This unnecessary tension not only causes a lot of discomfort but also acts as an enormous drain on our energy resources. It is a major cause of tiredness and ill health, because energy is being used both to tell the muscles to contract and to keep them contracted, even if we are only half aware of it. In this section we present the technique for proper relaxation, to which there are three aspects: the physical, the mental and the spiritual.

To relax the body, you lie down in the CORPSE POSE and first tense, then relax each part of the body in turn, working up from your feet to your head. This alternate tensing, then relaxing is necessary because it is only by knowing how tension feels that you can be sure that you have achieved relaxation. Then, just as in day-to-day life, your mind instructs the muscles to tense and contract, you now use auto-suggestion to send the muscles a message to relax. With practice you will gradually learn to use your subconscious mind to extend this control to the involuntary muscles of the heart, digestive system and other organs too.

To relax and focus the mind you breathe steadily and rhythmically and concentrate on your breathing. Mental and physical relaxation can never be complete, however, until you achieve spiritual peace. For as long as you identify with your body and mind, there will be fears and worries, anger and sorrow. Spiritual relaxation means detaching yourself, becoming a witness to the body and mind in order to identify with the self, or pure consciousness – the source of truth and peace that lies within us all.

In the course of relaxation you will feel sensations of melting down, of expansion, lightness and warmth. When all muscular tension is gone, a gentle euphoria suffuses the whole body. Relaxation is not so much a state as a process, a series of levels of increasing depth. It is a matter of letting go, instead of holding on; of not doing, rather than doing.

As you relax the whole body and breathe slowly and deeply, certain physiological changes occur: less oxygen is consumed and less carbon dioxide is eliminated; muscle tension is reduced; there is a decrease in the activity of the sympathetic nervous system – the involuntary system that mobilizes the instinctive responses, such as pupil dilation, increased heart rate, release of adrenalin and faster breathing, that arise from stress.

There is also an increase in parasympathetic activity from that part of the nervous system that works involuntarily to slow down the heart, calm the breath and promote relaxation. Even a few minutes of deep relaxation will reduce worry and fatigue more effectively than many hours of restless sleep.

3. RELAXATION AND GUIDED MEDITATION

PHYSICAL EFFECTS

The best time to practice relaxation and guided meditation is after completing a series of physical sequences. Your muscles will then be better toned and stretched and thus able to relax more fully. The postures in themselves help to bring your body and mind into a receptive state.

Relaxation brings down the heart rate, slows and deepens the breath and gently rests the body.

EMOTIONAL REFLECTIONS

Any accumulated worries and stresses will have been soothed by the physical workout, and calmness, relaxation and spiritual peace will follow from an already prepared state of being. The mind will slowly become clear and removed from everyday life.

MEDITATION
I am at peace, and I feel an integral part of the universe

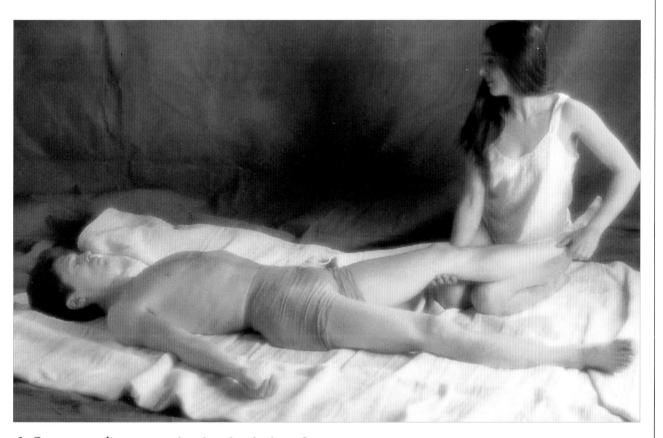

1. One partner lies on their back, flat on the floor; the other gently lifts and stretches each leg in turn, with one hand under the knee for support while they stretch out the back of the heels.

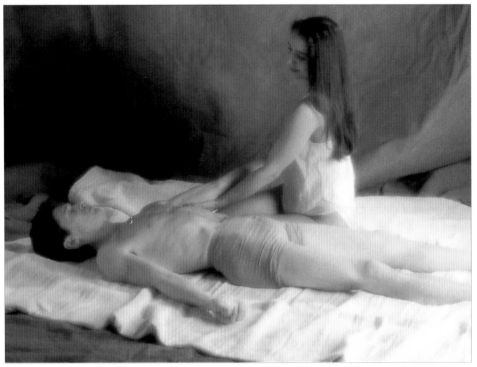

sinking down into the floor.

7. Feel your back and hips as heavy and sinking. Allow your whole body to release down into the floor and out into the space around you.

8. Focus your attention on the rise and fall of the breath. Let it come and go of its own accord with the abdomen rising slightly with the in-breath and falling with the out-breath. Allow any thoughts that come into your mind to float off with the breath, just feeling calm and still and very relaxed.

9. When the reclining partner is fully relaxed, the supporting partner sits comfortably and reads the guided meditation (page 78).

10. This reclining embrace is a sensual way to complete the meditation.

2. (above) Stretch out the arms and pull the shoulder-blades down and in by placing one hand underneath each shoulder-blade; lift and stretch the arm with the other hand by pulling from the wrist.

3. (opposite) Lift the head and take all the weight of it in the palms of your hands. Extend the head away from the shoulders and then gently rest the back of the head on the floor.

4. The prone partner looks up to the ceiling as high as possible without disturbing the position of the head. Allow the eyeballs to sink heavily down into their sockets as though looking deep into the body.

5. Relax the jaw by allowing the back teeth to fall away from each other. Relax and soften the throat, allow the tip of the tongue to rest on the upper palate.

6. Feel the heaviness of your arms and legs

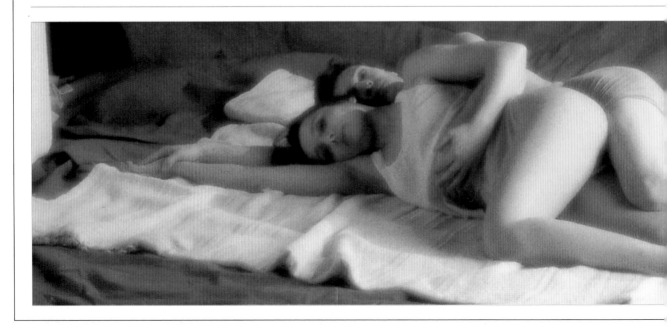

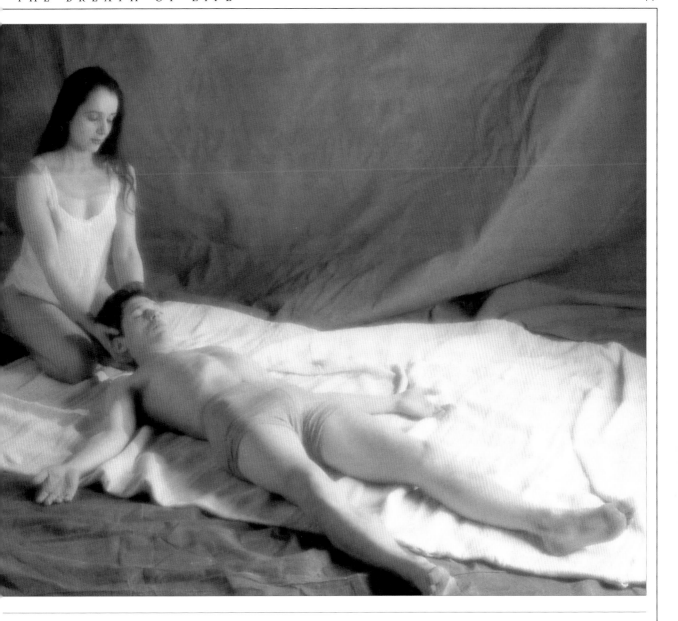

HELPFUL HINTS

• SEE IF YOU can let yourself go completely while relaxing. Think of the skin being soft and sensitive and then draw the energy away from the perimeters of your body.

• TAKE AS MUCH time as you need to release any discomfort in your body. If the lower back feels strained then bend the legs; take the knees together while keeping the feet slightly apart. Try to relax completely into the guided meditation.

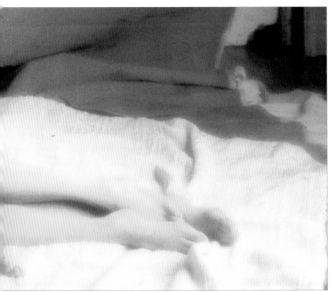

GUIDED MEDITATION

Take a deep breath and fill your chest with air. Let it expand your chest fully, so that you can feel the muscles stretch. Good. Now hold your breath for a moment. And release the air slowly, and allow your chest and shoulder muscles to relax, letting go. As the air flows out naturally and freely, feel the tension release in your muscles and inside yourself. Let the listening part of yourself focus on my voice as you feel yourself drifting into a state of relaxation. Feeling so peaceful, so light, so free of any tenseness. It is as if your whole self is released from pressure, permitting your natural energies to restore themselves and flow back into your body with new vigor for when you need it. Let yourself go deeper into this relaxed state.

Bring your attention to bear on your feet: from the toes and the arches, to the soles and the heels. Concentrate on the muscles of your feet. Very slowly begin to tighten them, so that the toes start to curl under, the arches rise. The tension increases from your toes to your heels. Take a deep breath and slowly release it. Let go, and slowly, gently, allow the muscles to relax, until all the tightness is gone. Let your feet relax totally, so that every bit of residual tension drains away. Take another deep breath. Let it go, and let the awareness of your feet fade away into a comfortable state of quietness, almost detached, so relaxed.

Now focus on the area from your ankles up to your knees. Feel the weight of your legs on the floor and slowly begin to tighten the muscles of your legs from your ankles to your knees. Bring these leg muscles to a peak of tension, and hold it there for a moment. Slowly allow the muscles to relax, letting go and releasing, until all of them are once again relaxed, free of tightness. Take a deep breath very slowly and hold it. Now slowly let it go, and, as you breathe out, shift the focus of awareness away from your legs. Let them drift out of the consciousness into a comfortable state of quietness, feeling somewhat detached, along with the feet. So relaxed. So released.

Focus your awareness on the area from your knees to your thighs, back to your buttocks and to

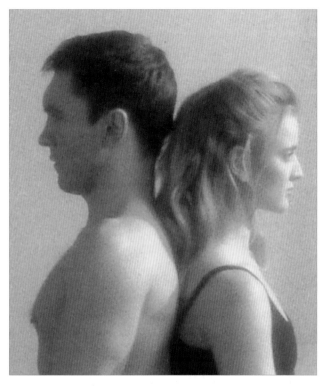

Let your whole body unwind and feel free, floating and relaxed

your lower back. Experience your weight as it presses down upon the floor, and the return pressure from the floor against the lower part of your back. Slowly and gently begin to make these muscles tense, from your knees, your thighs, your lower back and the whole pelvic area. Bring these muscles to a peak of tension. And hold it there for a moment. Gently allow these muscles to relax; let go and feel the thigh muscles let go too as the pelvis settles back on to the floor. Let all the muscles go loose. Take a deep breath, and hold it. As you very slowly let out the air, complete the muscle relaxation of your thighs and pelvis. Take a very deep breath. Hold it for a moment. As you let out your breath, allow your knees, thighs, pelvis and lower back to drift into a comfortable, quiet feeling. A dreamy, detached state. So quiet and so relaxed.

Focus your awareness on your chest, your upper body, your shoulders and your upper back. Become aware of the steady beating of your heart, of your lungs taking in and releasing air as you need it. Feel your back resting against the floor. Take a deep breath, drawing in the air slowly. Pull in the muscles of your stomach, expand your chest and raise it to its fullest. Tighten your shoulder muscles until all the muscles of the upper chest are at top tension. Hold it. Experience the full expansion. Now slowly let the air out of your chest. Let your stomach muscles relax, and your chest drop down. Press out all the air in your chest that is possible, then let go and feel yourself unwind throughout your upper body. Let your awareness move away from your upper body and allow the quiet and comfortable, detached and dreamy feeling to flow through your neck, your jaw, your cheek muscles, your forehead and your eye muscles.

Slowly tighten the muscles of your neck and jaw so that your teeth begin to clench. Let the muscles of your eyes, face and scalp tighten until a peak of tension is reached. Now allow them slowly to relax. Let your jaw muscles unlock. Your teeth unclench. Your scalp and face smooth out. Your jaw may release so much that it opens partially; just let it relax fully. Take a deep breath, and, as you exhale slowly, continue to let go. Allow your awareness of your head and neck to fade away. Let the detached, dreamy feeling drift all over your head and neck.

Focus your attention upon your fingers. Your hands. Your wrists. Your forearms. And your upper arms. Feel your hand slowly forming a fist as the fingers close up tightly. Let the muscles become more and more tense, until they reach a peak of tension. Hold it. Very slowly release and let your fingers unroll and your fist open. Allow your forearms and upper arms to relax and your arms to press lightly against the floor, so all the tension drains away. Your whole body unwinds fully, as the quiet, detached, dreamy feeling flows all through you, helping you to feel so floating, free and relaxed.

When you come out of this relaxation, do so carefully and slowly with no sudden movements. Rest quietly in the CHILD'S POSE for a while.

Pranayama

The fundamental effect of the practice of yoga is the nurturing of life force, or prana. Prana dwells in matter, but it is not material. It is a subtle form of energy that is carried in air, food, water and sunlight and animates all forms of matter. This energy is controlled by a combination of yoga asanas and 'pranayama', as yogic breathing is called.

In the yogic tradition prana is also the link between our physical and spiritual selves. Physically, pranayama takes in and stores in the body our life force, bringing greater vitality and strength. Spiritually, pranayama encourages kundalini, or cosmic energy, to rise through the seven chakras, or centers of energy, of our astral bodies. Raising the kundalini from the base chakra, or muladhara, to sahasrara, the highest chakra, means the yogi has achieved samadhi, or complete enlightenment, a level of existence beyond time, space and causation.

Yogic breathing, then, helps achieve physical well-being and spiritual enlightenment. Once you are familiar with SITTING BREATHING and LYING BREATHING, practice a more advanced breathing technique, Anuloma Viloma, or alternate-nostril breathing.

1. As in SITTING BREATHING raise your right hand, close the right nostril with the thumb and exhale completely through the left nostril.
2. Inhale completely through the left nostril, keeping the right nostril closed.
3. Close both nostrils and hold the breath for a few seconds.
4. Release the right nostril and exhale slowly and completely.
5. Inhale fully through the right nostril.
6. Close both nostrils and retain the breath for a few seconds.

Try to repeat this exercise several times, gradually building up to ten complete cycles.

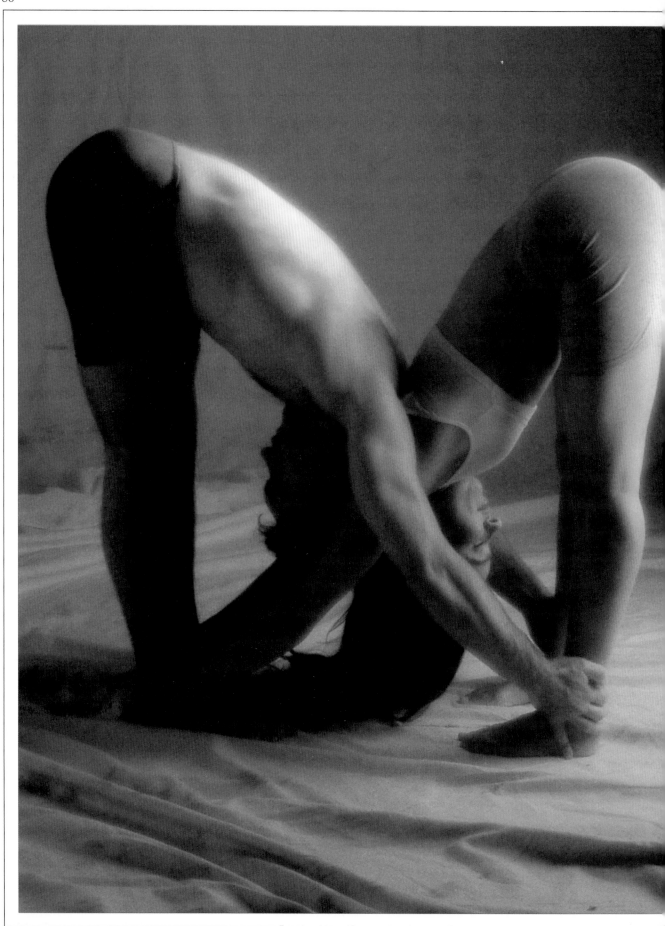

RELEASING THE DAY TOGETHER

STRESS CAN BE A POSITIVE FORCE. Without it there is little drive, motivation or challenge. As pressure increases, so does our performance. We enjoy the demands made on us. Stress triggers the energy to create and achieve as well as to survive.

Love requires only opening and trusting.
When everything is opened and released, then
there is love.

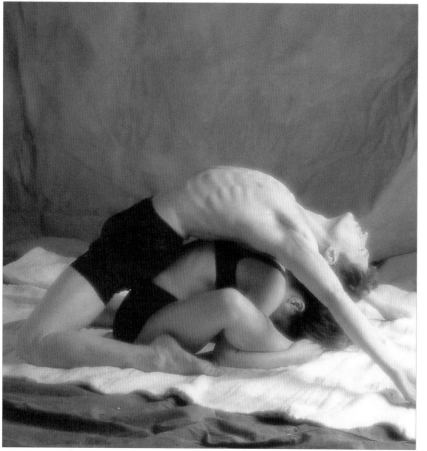

Intimate touch and support release tension

sion in the muscles and make it difficult for us to get the good night's sleep essential to set us up for the next day and prevent more stress accumulation.

There are many forms of stress relief on offer. Clever marketing convinces us of the need for external remedies – whether in the form of pills, alcohol or therapy. In fact very many of life's crises can be successfully surmounted without resorting to any external remedies. Helping ourselves from our own resources makes us stronger and better able to cope the next time. Reaching for unnecessary stimulants and tranquillizers is weakening and breeds dependence.

With a little time and patience we can alleviate stress, in all its different forms. We may be powerless to solve the problems, but we can certainly do a great deal to prevent them from overwhelming us. It may take surprisingly little to brighten our outlook.

For a start we can reverse the syndrome of physical tensions caused by emotional setbacks or hostile circumstances. The sequences in this chapter will exercise the body and improve breathing, allowing us to take in more oxygen to nourish our body and brain, helping us to respond constructively to the stress around us. It is less likely that we will stockpile the negative aspects of stress in the course of our day if our bodies and minds are open and strong.

The intimate touch and support involved in these sequences is the ideal way to release and relax these stored tensions. In time we shall observe a new depth in our relationship; a deeper sensitivity to each other's needs and weaknesses. The practice of *The Art of Sensual Yoga* at the end of the day will help provide some punctuation between our day's work and our time together. It will help to bring us back to each other.

But we also know that too much stress is harmful. We are all familiar with the days when the telephone never stops ringing, when the home or office seems to demand reserves that we do not feel we possess. By the end of such a day we may be exhausted, yet not able to calm down. We may become irritable, not finding it possible to relax, our body tired and tight with fatigue. In these circumstances we may experience the effects of stress but not the release through the physical action that our body expects to follow the tension. As frustration builds up, each crisis makes an overstressed person more vulnerable.

We perhaps do not often express anger and anxiety openly with our body. Instead we are more likely to repress irritation and react to the frustrations that accumulate in the course of a day by tightening our muscles. If we end a working day full of resentment and aggression, we cannot get going again properly until we have got rid of our negative feelings. These are stored as ten-

1. CALMING

PHYSICAL EFFECTS

This is a wonderful sequence for you and your partner to perform together at the end of a busy day. It will help to release accumulated stiffness and tension from your whole body. You will feel in a relaxed frame of mind for the evening ahead.

The sitting position provides a good stretch for the thighs and the ankles, and the upward stretch is wonderful for extending the spine and for relieving stiffness in the shoulders. The abdominal organs are toned and the arms well stretched. The chest is opened fully, and thus the capacity to breathe deeply is increased.

It is a particularly suitable sequence for you to do together as it is hard to achieve full stretch on one's own. This sequence is quite powerful if time is taken really to release into it. See if you can feel yourself slowly letting go as you stretch, giving your body time to experience the effects fully, without strain.

This sequence is a good prelude to further workouts in the chapter as the legs, spine and chest will be toned and open, ready to move on to the more demanding sequences.

EMOTIONAL REFLECTIONS

This sequence has been developed to release stiffness in the shoulders and neck, where the stresses of the day are stored. It also quiets the mind, allowing you to feel peaceful and relaxed.

MEDITATION
I allow peace and calm into my life

1. Sit on your heels, one behind the other.

2. Place your hands on the partner in front's shoulders, gently drawing them down. Make sure the tailbone tucks under, the buttocks sink down and the chest lifts.

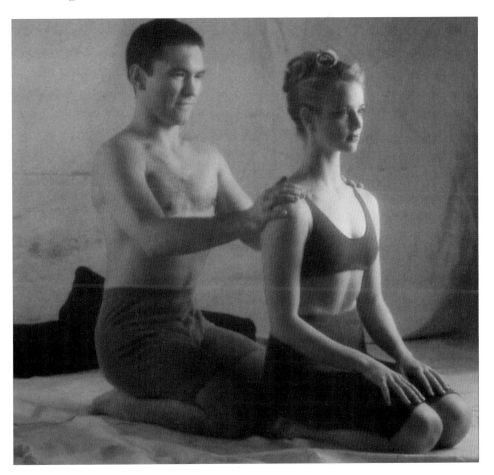

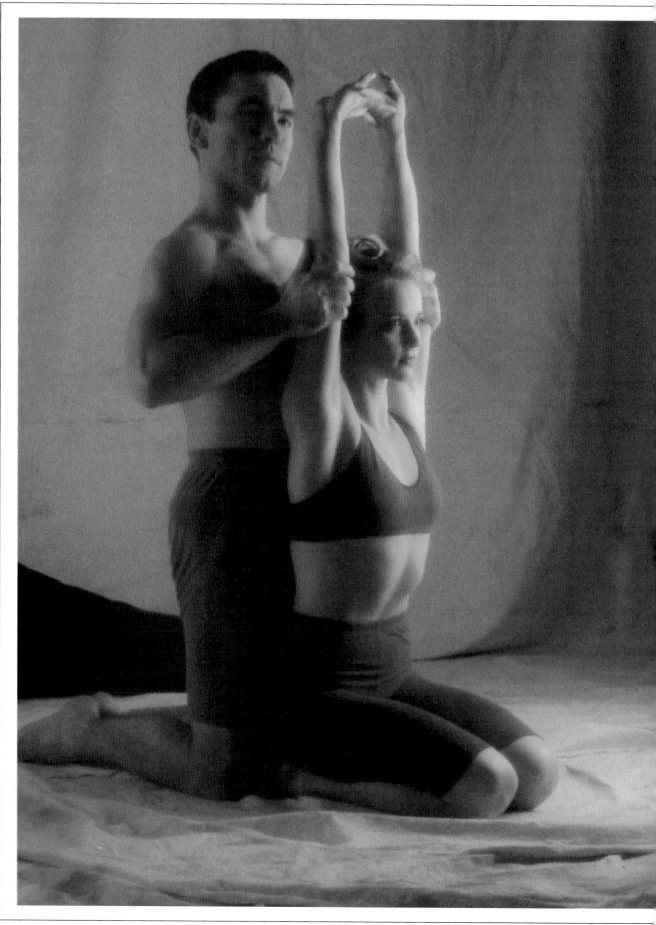

3. (left) The partner in front interlaces their fingers, turns their palms upward and stretches up. At the same time move the lower spine in without pushing the front ribs forward, then lift the diaphragm as you stretch up, keeping the spine extended.

4. The supporting partner helps the up-stretch by drawing the arms up and away from the shoulders.

5. Keeping the throat soft and jaw relaxed, now stretch up and up, feeling the back ribs lifting away from the waist. Hold the stretch for four to five breaths.

6. Release the grip, bring your arms down and interlace the palms with the opposite thumb on top. Hold for four to five breaths.

7. Release the grip and stretch both arms down towards the floor for a few breaths.

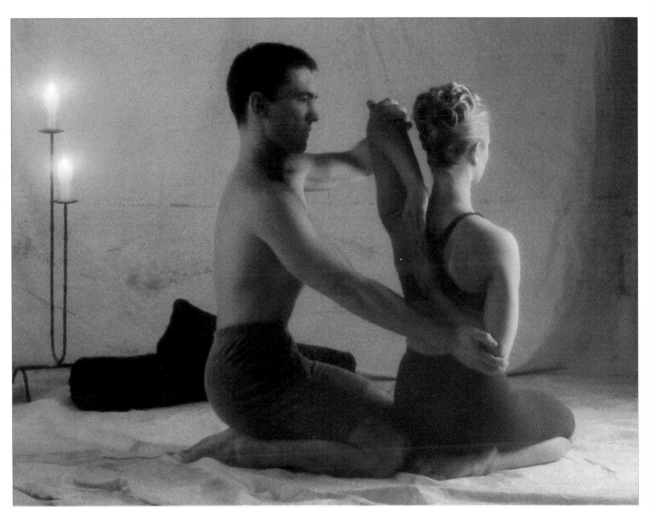

8. Now stretch the left arm up, hold the stretch for a few breaths while taking the right hand up in between the shoulderblades. Bend the left arm at the elbow and catch the right hand.

9. The supporting partner helps the extension of the left arm up by drawing it back so that it is in line with the left ear, at the same time keeping the right elbow back and down. Stretch the back of your neck away from the spine. Hold the grip for four to five breaths.

10. Release the grip and repeat the movement on the other side. Hold for four to five breaths.

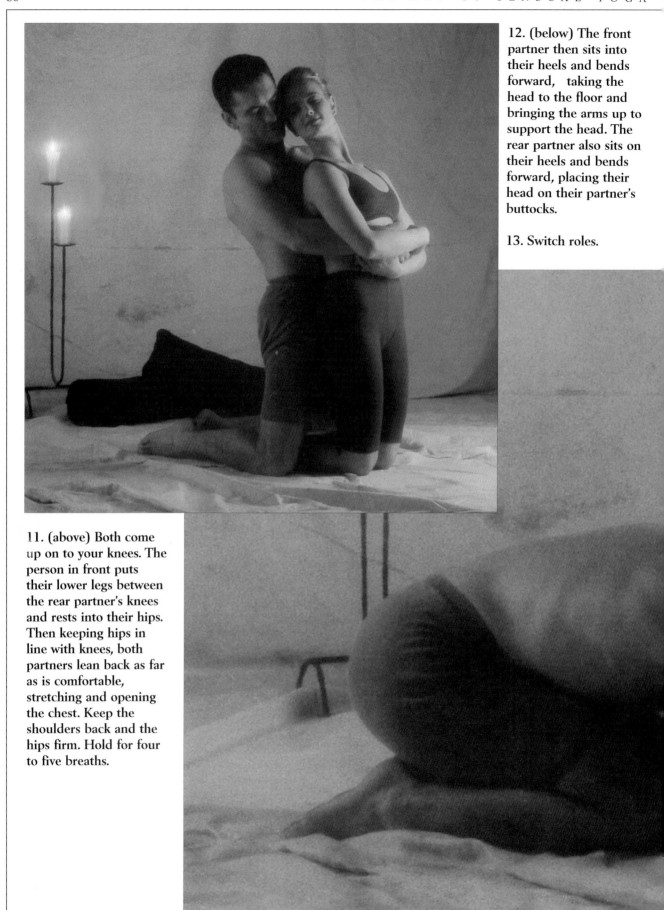

12. (below) The front partner then sits into their heels and bends forward, taking the head to the floor and bringing the arms up to support the head. The rear partner also sits on their heels and bends forward, placing their head on their partner's buttocks.

13. Switch roles.

11. (above) Both come up on to your knees. The person in front puts their lower legs between the rear partner's knees and rests into their hips. Then keeping hips in line with knees, both partners lean back as far as is comfortable, stretching and opening the chest. Keep the shoulders back and the hips firm. Hold for four to five breaths.

HELPFUL HINTS

• IF SITTING ON the heels proves uncomfortable, then the arm-raising parts of the sequence can be done from a cross-legged position, with one partner kneeling behind.

• TAKE PLENTY OF time with the different stages of the sequence. If you are stiff in the shoulders and cannot grip the wrists behind the back, then hold a belt between the hands to help to maximize the stretch.

• AS USUAL KEEP the face relaxed and breathe in as you stretch into the posture and out as you release through it.

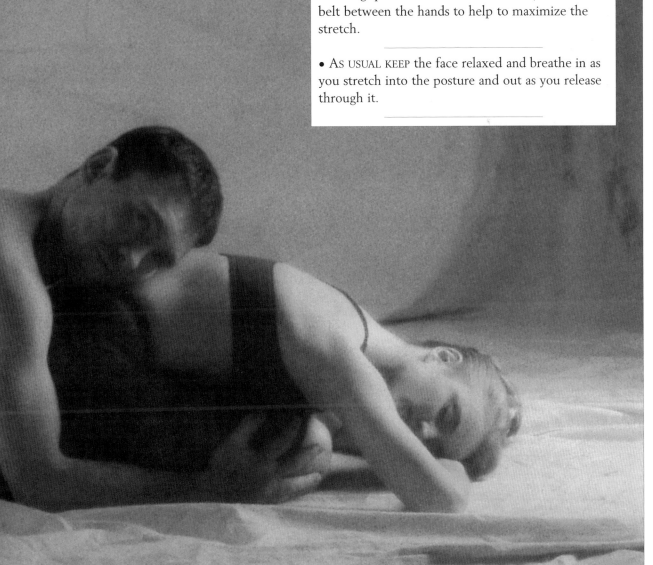

2. GATHERING

PHYSICAL EFFECTS

In this sequence the spine is strongly stretched, and tension in the lower back is released if the movements are performed slowly and with care.

The shoulders are stretched and the chest fully opened. The thighs are also stretched and toned.

The stomach is stretched and toned, so gastric problems can be relieved.

The support of your partner will help you to take the stretch to your own limit, thus gaining maximum benefit from the sequence.

EMOTIONAL REFLECTIONS

At the end of the day our energies are often scattered. This uplifting sequence gathers us together, encouraging us to focus and center ourselves. It is uplifting and restorative.

MEDITATION

I am safe in the world. I have gathered my power into its proper place

1. One partner lies front down on the floor with their supportive partner kneeling beside them, gently stretching their arms away from their shoulders.

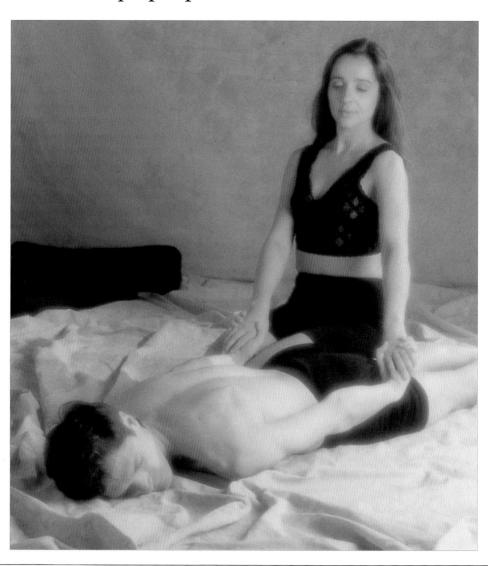

2. The reclining partner interlaces their fingers, palms facing their back. The helping partner gently stretches the arms back, the chest lifts off the floor. Press the hips into the floor and stretch the legs back firmly. Keeping buttocks taut, tailbone down towards the floor, tuck the shoulder-blades into the back and lift the chest even higher. The arms follow the line from the shoulders throughout. Hold for four to five breaths.

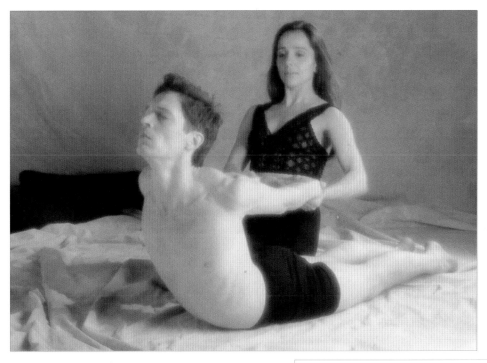

LOCUST POSE
(*Sanskrit*: Salabhasana)

'SALABHA' MEANS 'LOCUST', AND THIS POSE APPARENTLY RESEMBLES THE GRASSHOPPER-LIKE INSECT AS IT RESTS ON THE GROUND. THE ASANA HELPS TO RELIEVE GASTRIC PROBLEMS AND AIDS THE DIGESTIVE SYSTEM. THE SPINE IS WELL EXERCISED, AND THE POSITION CAN HELP TO ALLEVIATE PAIN IN THE SACRAL AND LUMBAR REGIONS.

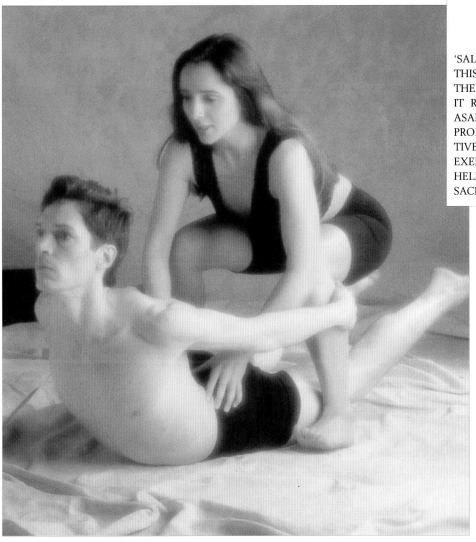

3. The supportive partner squats, feet either side of the prone partner, who catches the helper's lower legs; while the helper pushes the tailbone down, the prone partner lifts and stretches their legs back into the LOCUST POSE.

4. The prone partner keeps the buttocks firm throughout, lifting the collar-bones and extending through the spine and neck.

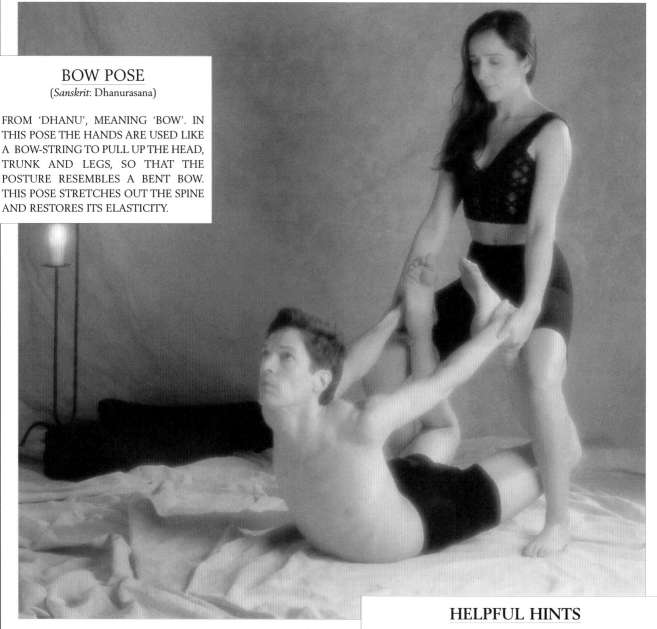

BOW POSE
(*Sanskrit*: Dhanurasana)

FROM 'DHANU', MEANING 'BOW'. IN THIS POSE THE HANDS ARE USED LIKE A BOW-STRING TO PULL UP THE HEAD, TRUNK AND LEGS, SO THAT THE POSTURE RESEMBLES A BENT BOW. THIS POSE STRETCHES OUT THE SPINE AND RESTORES ITS ELASTICITY.

5. Rest for a minute or two.
6. Then the prone partner goes into the BOW POSE by firmly catching hold of their ankles and drawing the knees and chest up. Their partner assists by catching hold of their wrists and ankles, helping to draw them up so the ribs and pelvic bones lift off the floor. Hold for four to five breaths.
7. Change roles.

HELPFUL HINTS

• THE ABDOMEN IS strongly extended in this sequence, so the breath will be short and fast. Still try to hold the poses for a minimum of four to five breaths in order to gain full benefit.

• IF THE PELVIS feels uncomfortable on the floor, place a folded blanket beneath the hips.

• AVOID STRAINING THE neck in this pose. Let the stretch work its way through your body rather than lifting with the neck, which is something we tend to do in these strong sequences.

• REMEMBER: THROAT, JAW and eyes soft.

3. FREEDOM

PHYSICAL EFFECTS

This is a well-balanced, gradually intensifying sequence. In the beginning the chest is gently opened, and the neck is extended without strain. By the end stages both the neck and chest are prepared for the stronger demands of the BRIDGE and BOW.

The BRIDGE POSE, as well as opening the chest strongly, gives a strong upward stretch to the thighs; the kidneys are toned, and the thyroid gland in the neck is stimulated.

The final part of the sequence is an intense stretch that takes the chest opening a stage further. The whole body then becomes involved in this strong upward lift, which is enhanced by the firm support of your partner.

Your nervous system will be toned by the intense stretch to the spine.

EMOTIONAL REFLECTIONS

This entire sequence works the whole body: it is extremely invigorating, frees tension and releases emotions. On resting you will feel completely energized, calm and clear-minded. Your spirits will be light and joyful.

MEDITATION
I free my body and allow my spirit to fly

1. Lie down on your back with your knees bent and your feet hip distance apart. Stretch your arms out on the floor beside your body. Your partner stands over you, feet either side of your head, supporting your back ribs.

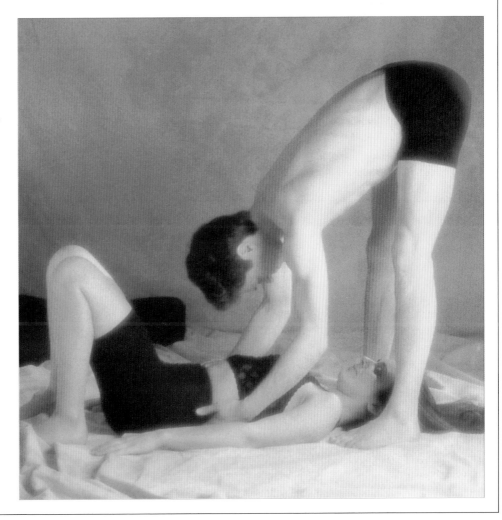

2. The supporting partner gently raises the reclining partner's back ribs while they keep the back of their head on the floor. Stretch your arms out in line with your shoulders and take your breastbone up towards your partner's face. Tuck your shoulder-blades into your back, relax your throat and breathe softly for four to five breaths.

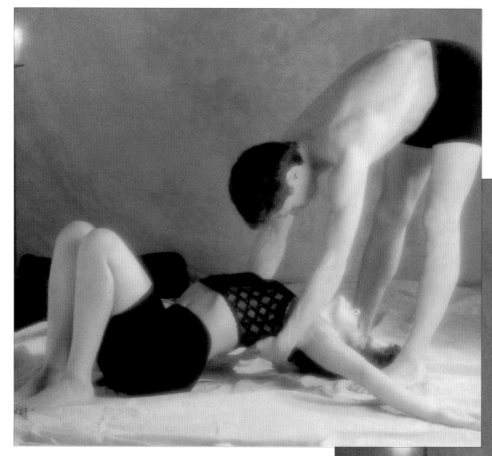

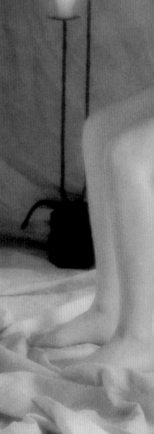

3. Lie flat and rest for a few seconds. Then push into your feet and lift up your hips, extending the tailbone away from your waist so as not to strain the lower back. Your partner supports your lower back and helps you lift even more. Lift your breastbone up and towards your partner's face. Tuck your shoulder-blades under your back, relax your throat and extend the back of your neck. Hold for four to five breaths.

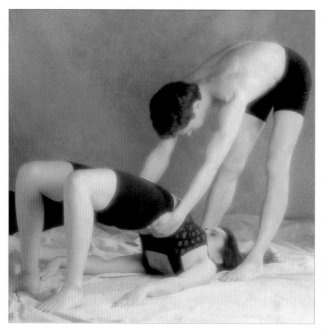

4. Catch hold of your partner's ankles and with their hands supporting your back lift up on top of your head. If you feel you can take the extension further, ask your partner to support you by placing their palms on your shoulders and draw you towards them while you stretch and straighten your arms and extend your tailbone up and away from them. However far you go in this sequence, hold the maximum stretch for four to five breaths.

THE BRIDGE
(*Sanskrit*: Setu Bandha Sarvaganasana)

THE BRIDGE STRETCHES THE SPINE AND RELAXES THE NECK. ITS SANSKRIT NAME MEANS 'BRIDGE-BUILDING POSE', REFERRING TO THE WAY IN WHICH THE BODY CREATES A PERFECT ARCH FROM HEAD TO TOE. MOVING INTO AND OUT OF THE POSITION STRENGTHENS THE ABDOMINAL AND LOWER-BACK MUSCLES AND MAKES THE SPINE AND WRISTS MORE SUPPLE.

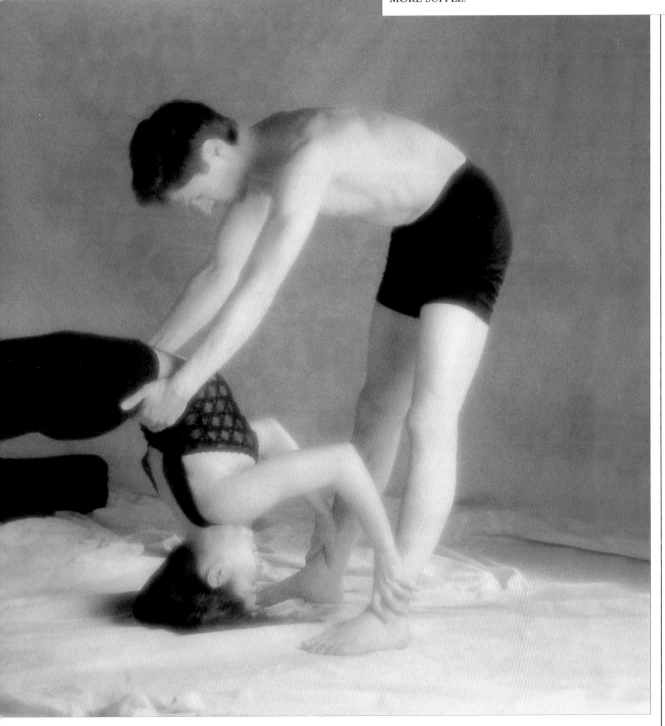

5. If you feel you can safely extend further, come up on to your toes. Walk your feet in a little and place your heels firmly back on the floor. Extend the lift of your chest towards your partner and your hips towards the ceiling. Hold for four to five breaths.

6. (below) Return to the first position with the gentle assistance of your partner. Sit up in COBBLER POSE and bend forward, touching your head to the floor if possible. Your partner sits just below the rim of the pelvis and leans back along your spine, while taking their feet beside your hips and stretching their arms out to the side. Remain in this position for at least 30 seconds.

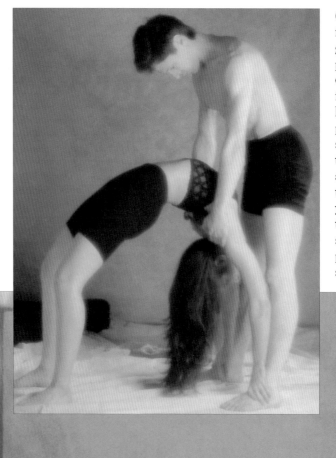

HELPFUL HINTS

• PLENTY OF TIME needs to be taken to complete this demanding sequence safely. Pause after each stage and be aware of the limits of your flexibility.

• IF AT ANY time during the sequence you feel that you have stretched enough, then come back to the resting position.

• KEEP THE FEET very firm in the lifting part of the sequence and in line with the shins. Avoid turning the feet out to the sides.

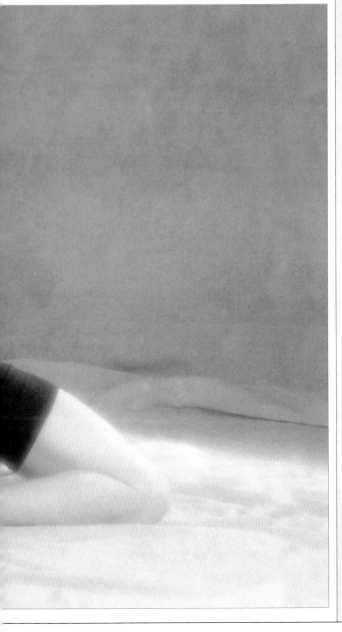

Yoga as exercise

Increasingly in the English-speaking world yoga is becoming popular as a form of physical exercise. Initially people often practiced yoga as a compliment to other kinds of exercise, such as aerobics, weight training or other sports. But now yoga is considered more and more seriously as a complete form of exercise in its own right.

Most serious athletes these days employ yoga-based asanas as part of their training, which, at the most basic level, helps improve flexibility while maintaining strength. Yogic exercises are also very good at encouraging shortened muscles to stretch. Athletes have recognized that improved strength, flexibility and mobility in the joints and musculature reduce the incidence and seriousness of injuries. Improvements in cardiovascular efficiency have also been observed.

Most of us, of course, are not athletes and may exercise only once or twice a week at aerobic classes or workouts. However, the benefits of yoga are equally as effective. In addition to all its physical benefits there is one important element that elevates yoga above all other types of exercise: the mind factor.

The power of yoga is its ability to bring the body to a state of effortless poise and the mind to a point of stillness. This change of consciousness reflects the experience of total unity, which allows us to be in touch with what yogis call the higher universal self.

In effect yoga provides a form of complete mind/body meditation: through exercise one stills the mind and enters into a timeless state of heightened awareness and total concentration in the present moment.

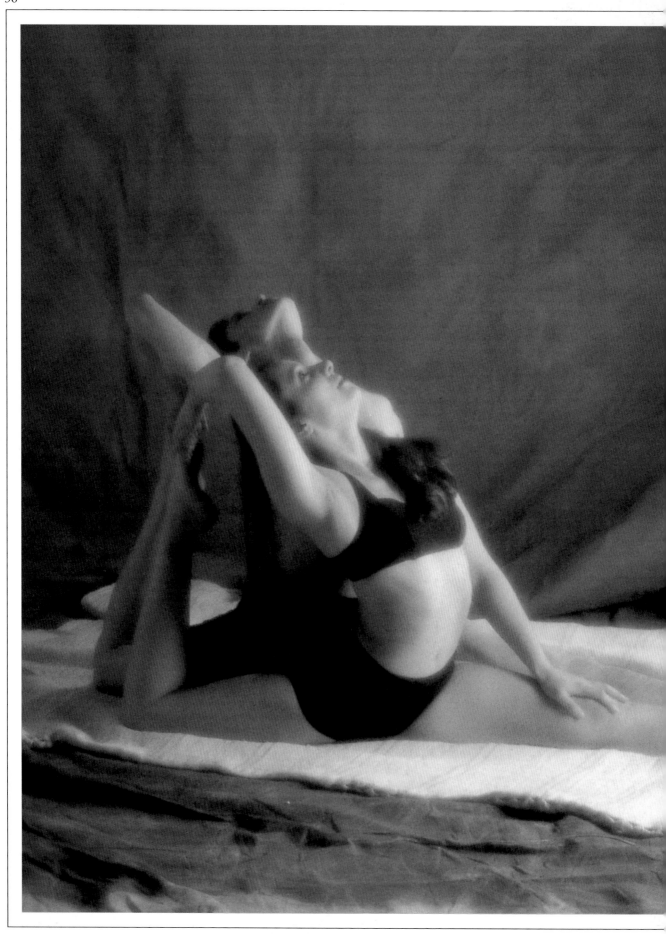

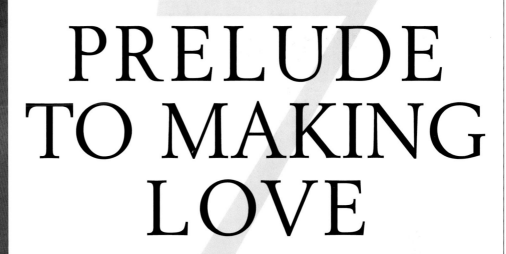

PRELUDE TO MAKING LOVE

Love is an active power, a force that breaks through the walls that separate, uniting us one with the other. The art of loving overcomes our sense of isolation and separateness, and yet permits us to be ourselves, to retain our integrity. Mature love is union under the condition of preserving our individuality.

Love is rhythmic. It moves like tides and seasons. Lovers fill each other with the rhythm of life.

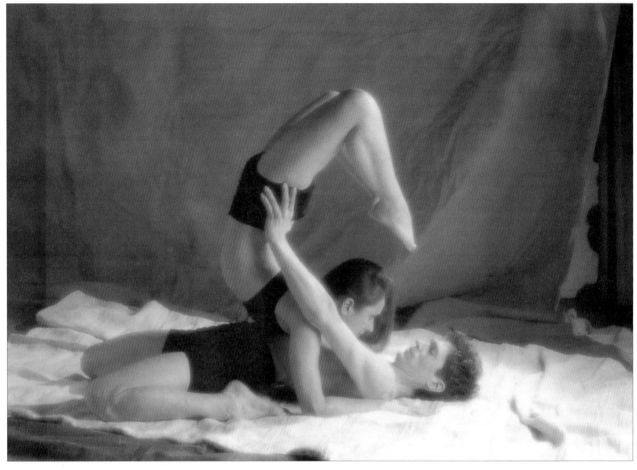

It is through erotic love that we experience ourselves as alive and joyous

Love is an activity, not a passive effect. The art of loving is primarily to give, not to receive. At its highest level giving has an entirely different meaning. It involves not giving up, or sacrificing, but an exchange. Through love we gain a strength and vitality that fills us with joy. We experience ourselves as overflowing, alive and joyous. Giving is more joyous than receiving, because in the act of giving there is no deprivation, simply an expression of our aliveness.

The most elementary example of this is seen in the sphere of sexual love. The culmination of the male sexual drive lies in the act of giving. The man gives himself, his sexual organ, to the woman. At the moment of orgasm he presents his semen to her. He cannot help doing so! For the woman the process is no different, although more complex. She gives herself, too, as she opens the gates to her feminine center; in the act of receiving, she gives.

In this process of fusion a couple begin to know themselves. They learn by the experience of union. Erotic love is the need for complete fusion. It has one premise: love from the essence of our being – with a parallel experience of the other person in the essence of their being. It is an explosive engagement, with a sudden collapse of barriers.

The yoga sequences that follow have been developed to help us, as couples, to experience the full power of erotic love and to counter the effects that distracted, stressful life-styles can have on our relationships. The philosophy behind these sequences is to allow us to enjoy intimate physical and emotional contact together without any pressure to make love. The prelude to erotic love is the development of certain basic elements, common to all forms of love: care, responsibility, respect and knowledge – active concern for the life of those whom we love. Only by working on these basic elements can we give ourselves to the power of erotic love.

1. NURTURING

It is suggested that Calming, the first sequence from chapter 6, 'Releasing the Day Together', is completed before embarking on the first movements of this chapter.

PHYSICAL EFFECTS
The next two sequences will open up the whole body with a good stretch, before embarking on the more strenuous SHOULDER STAND, followed by the relaxing sequence at the end of the chapter.

With your partner's support you will feel able to give yourself fully to the stretch and find it possible to hold the strong lift for longer. Nurturing provides a wonderful stretch for the whole body, while strengthening the arms and wrists at the same time.

The shoulder joints are released and strengthened, while the chest is fully opened.

EMOTIONAL REFLECTIONS
The support of your partner is essential in Nurturing to awaken your sexual and emotional centers: the hips, buttocks, groin and chest. You will begin to feel more sexually aware.

MEDITATION
Your support nurtures and cares for me

1. Sit across your partner's thighs. Allow them to support you by holding your waist and thighs. Keep your arms in line with your shoulders and hands on the floor.

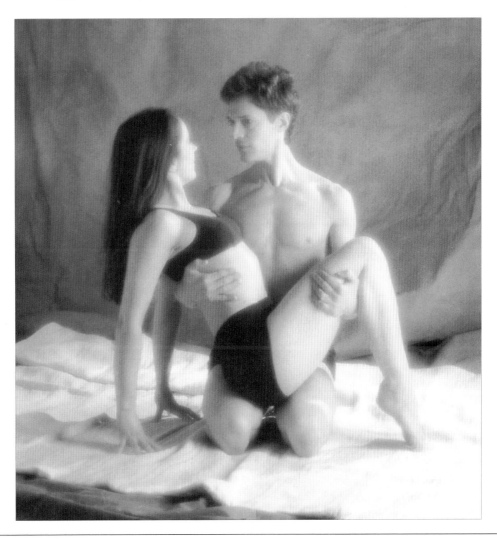

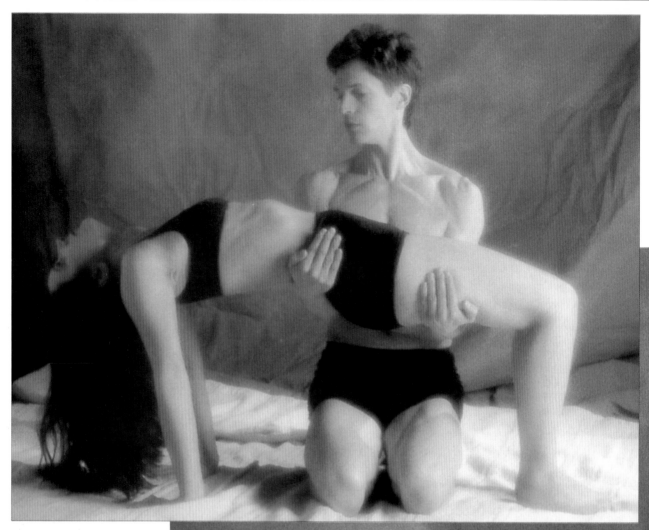

2. (above) Your partner
then lifts your hips so
that they align with your
shoulders. Hold for four
to five breaths.

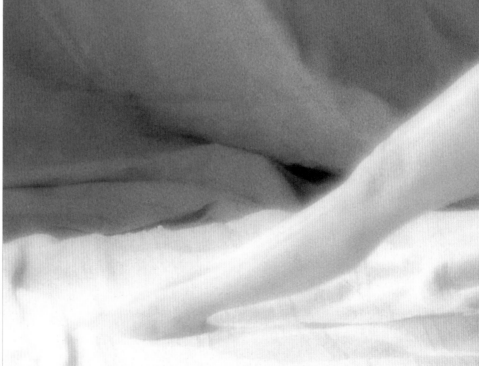

3. Straighten out your legs and stretch fully into them; keep your feet extending evenly towards the floor. Stretch your head back, with the shoulder-blades still tucked in. The middle of your thighs are facing up towards the ceiling, your insteps turned down towards the floor. Your hips are lifting up strongly and tailbone moving in and up towards the pubis. Your partner supports your lower back with both hands and forearms. Hold for four to five breaths.

4. Your partner gently lowers you to the floor. Lean forward in COBBLER POSE to counterstretch your spine.

5. Switch roles.

HELPFUL HINTS

• IF THERE IS any strain in the neck during the sequence, focus on lengthening your neck into the base of the skull.

• BY KEEPING THE shoulder-blades well in and the collar-bones lifted, tension in the neck should release.

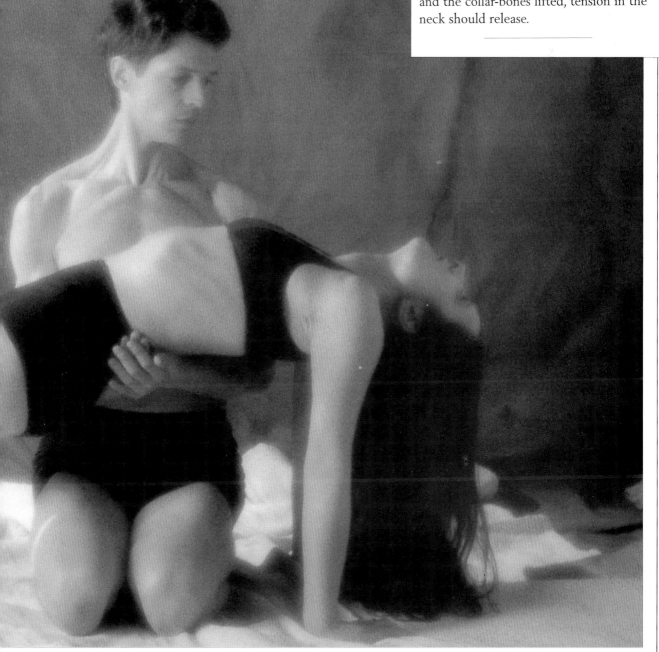

2. TOGETHERNESS

PHYSICAL EFFECTS

In Togetherness the body is already stretched and toned, and both partners can benefit simultaneously. It is an uplifting sequence to do with your partner's support as you can feel the slow opening and release in the chest and the freedom to breathe more fully while being supported.

This simple back bend helps to free stiff shoulders, open up the chest and firm the thighs. The kidneys are raised and toned.

In the final part of the sequence you will feel a wonderful stretch as you take your arms back and give your whole being to the pose.

EMOTIONAL REFLECTIONS

Allow your bodies to move together, holding and caressing each other. You stretch in harmony, each reflecting the other's movements in a dance of love.

MEDITATION
We are at peace with each other

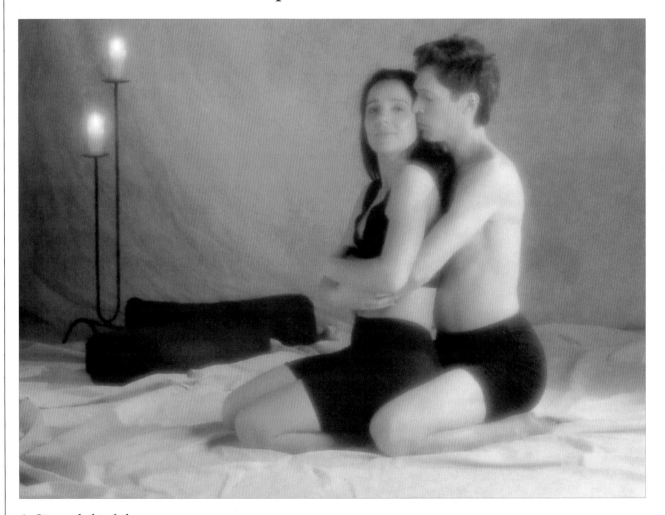

1. Sit one behind the other, with your hips resting on your feet.

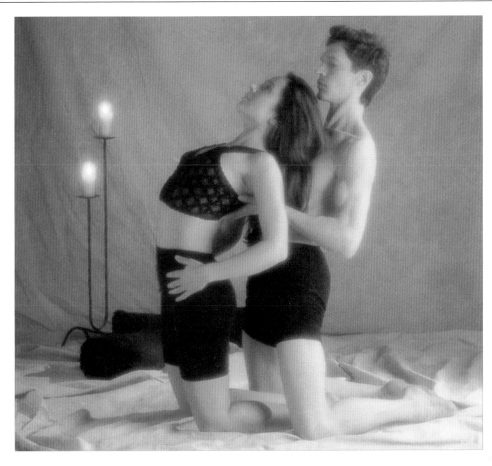

2. Both come up on to your knees, with your feet slightly apart and thighs perpendicular. Grip your hips and buttocks firmly, extending your ribs up and away from your hips while keeping your tailbones forward. Take your shoulder-blades into your backs. Stretch your abdomens up and lift your collar-bones. Focus on extending your necks into the base of your skulls. The supporting partner gently helps to lift their partner's back ribs, while they extend the back of their head towards the chest. Hold for four to five breaths.

3. Both lift your chests. The supporting partner places their hands on the front partner's hips, and both partners lean back, stretching their chests, tucking shoulder-blades in, lengthening their necks. The front partner places their hands on the supporting partner's. Hold for four to five breaths.

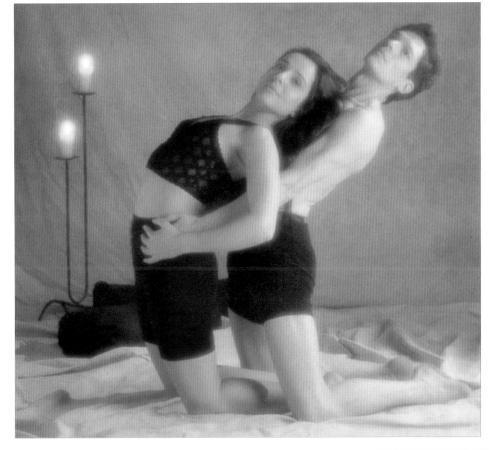

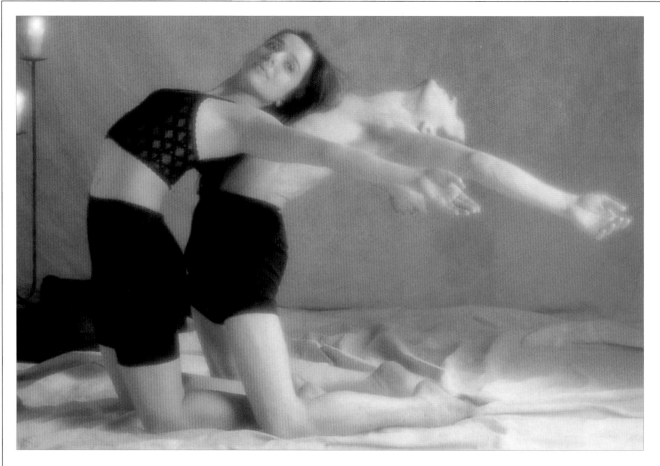

4. Both partners lean back fully into the pose, reaching their arms back and to the sides, stretching into their palms, extending their spines and chests. Hold for four to five breaths.

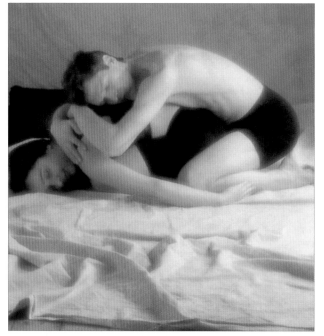

5. Lift forward and come down on to your knees. Bend forward, the supporting partner now stretching over the other partner's spine.

Relax in this pose and breathe deeply for a minute or two.

6 Switch roles.

HELPFUL HINTS

• PLACE A FOLDED blanket under the knees if they feel uncomfortable.

• IF THERE IS a feeling of tightness in the throat, make sure that the shoulder-blades are lifting well into the chest; that the collar-bones are lifting rather than the throat; that there is an extension in the base of the skull.

3. BALANCE

PHYSICAL EFFECTS

The SHOULDER STAND is one of the most important of the yoga postures. By inverting the body at right angles to the neck, the thyroids and parathyroids are stimulated. These are important glands in the neck, and with the firm chin-lock the blood supply is increased.

Because of the healthy blood supply circulating around the chest and neck, this sequence aids the healing of illnesses such as asthma, bronchitis and various throat ailments.

The posture also has a soothing effect on the nerves. The inner organs are nourished due to the inverted position, and constipation is relieved.

The circulation is improved as the venous blood returns to the heart without any strain.

You should try to hold the SHOULDER STAND for several minutes, so the support and help of your partner will be appreciated. After completing the sequence your whole body should be nourished and calm, and you will feel in tune with your partner.

EMOTIONAL REFLECTIONS

The SHOULDER STAND promotes emotional balance and stability. The support of your partner allows you to experience total freedom of your emotions.

MEDITATION

I am centered and freely give myself to you

1. Lie flat on the floor with your arms outstretched. Your partner stands with their feet either side of your hips and draws your lifted legs up towards them. Let your back release into the floor, extend your neck and relax your facial muscles.

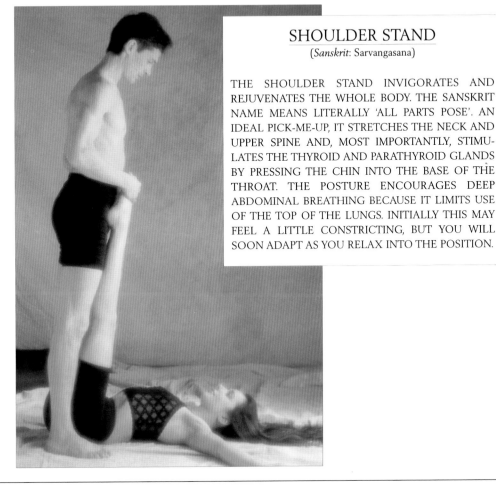

SHOULDER STAND
(*Sanskrit*: Sarvangasana)

THE SHOULDER STAND INVIGORATES AND REJUVENATES THE WHOLE BODY. THE SANSKRIT NAME MEANS LITERALLY 'ALL PARTS POSE'. AN IDEAL PICK-ME-UP, IT STRETCHES THE NECK AND UPPER SPINE AND, MOST IMPORTANTLY, STIMULATES THE THYROID AND PARATHYROID GLANDS BY PRESSING THE CHIN INTO THE BASE OF THE THROAT. THE POSTURE ENCOURAGES DEEP ABDOMINAL BREATHING BECAUSE IT LIMITS USE OF THE TOP OF THE LUNGS. INITIALLY THIS MAY FEEL A LITTLE CONSTRICTING, BUT YOU WILL SOON ADAPT AS YOU RELAX INTO THE POSITION.

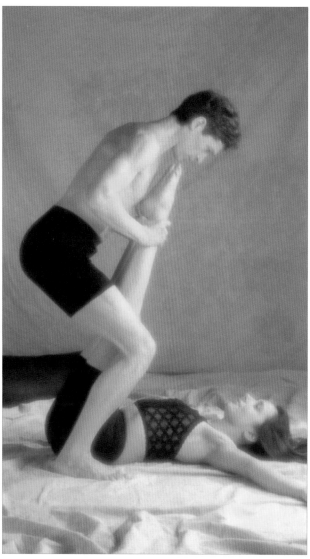

4. The reclining partner then supports their own back with the palms of their hands, while the standing partner goes around to the head and draws the legs up again. The reclining partner then releases the hold on their back and reaches for the standing partner's ankles.

2. (above) The standing partner then bends their legs and takes the reclining partner's legs by the ankles, lifting them up and stretching them out, drawing them slightly towards the reclining partner's face.

3. The standing partner then lifts the reclining partner on to their shoulders. The thighs support their hips and their legs stretch up to the chest. Only the back of the neck, head, shoulders and arms should be in contact with the floor, the remainder of the body, as much as possible, should be in a straight, upward line. Hold this pose for up to five minutes.

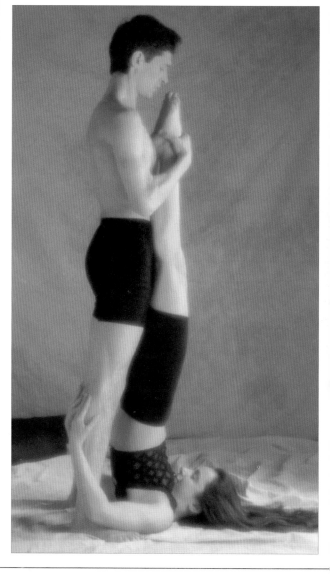

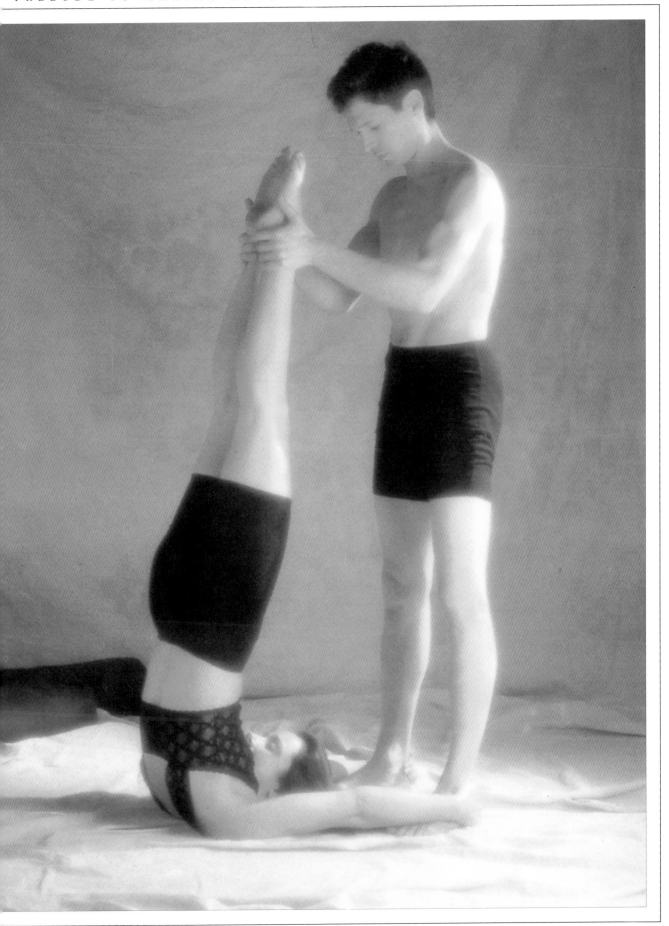

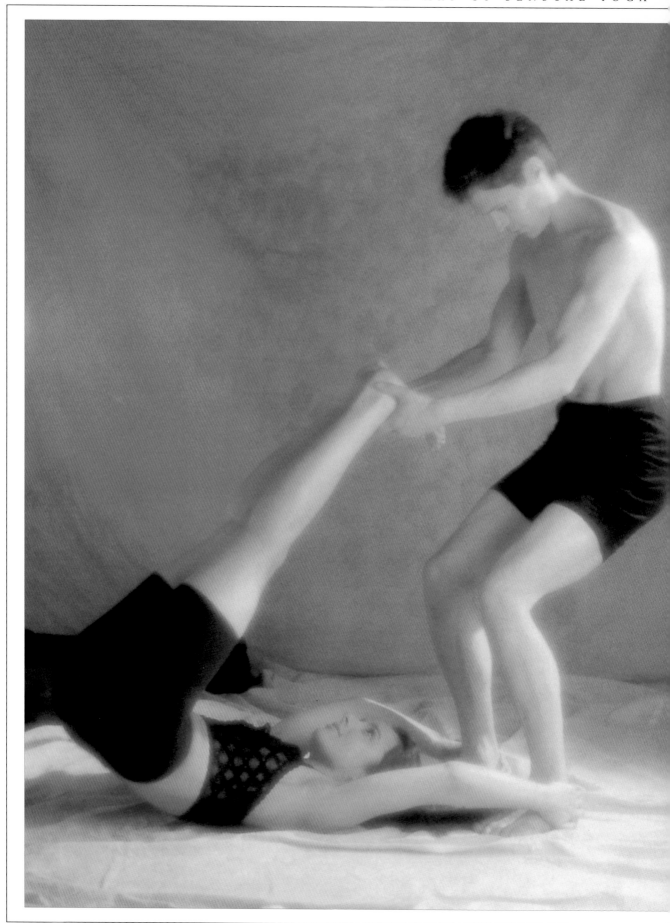

5. The standing partner then gradually lowers the reclining partner down on to their back, vertebra by vertebra.

HELPFUL HINTS

• DON'T DO THE SHOULDER STAND while menstruating. It is not considered good practice to invert the pelvis at this time.

• IF YOUR NECK feels strained in this pose, or if you feel pressure in your eyes, ears or throat, then allow your partner to ease you out of it slightly. Stretch the neck, and then see how you feel before you attempt to go into the full pose again. If you go up again and it still feels like a strain, then come down and go no further.

• SEE IF YOU can involve every part of your body in the pose. Lift, stretch and release. Make sure your throat, eyes and jaw remain passive.

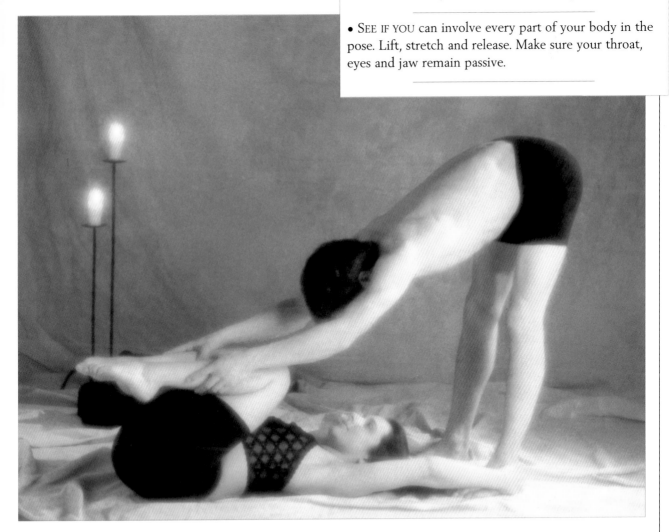

6. The reclining partner then takes their knees to their chest, as a counter-stretch, while the standing partner presses their partner's shins down into their thighs.

7. Switch roles.

4. EMBRACING

PHYSICAL EFFECTS

On a practical level, sitting and lying in this soft version of the COBBLER POSE relieves prostate, bladder and menstrual problems.

This sequence releases and relaxes the hips, thighs and abdomen: those parts of the body that are very much a part of the act of making love.

This soft and most sensual of poses provides an appropriate finale to the preceding sequences in the chapter. Your body will be toned, open and ready for love.

EMOTIONAL REFLECTIONS

By giving to each other in this way you can open yourselves to the power of love, to a feeling of complete abandonment with each other. There will be a feeling of spiritual, mental and physical integration between you.

MEDITATION
We are at one together

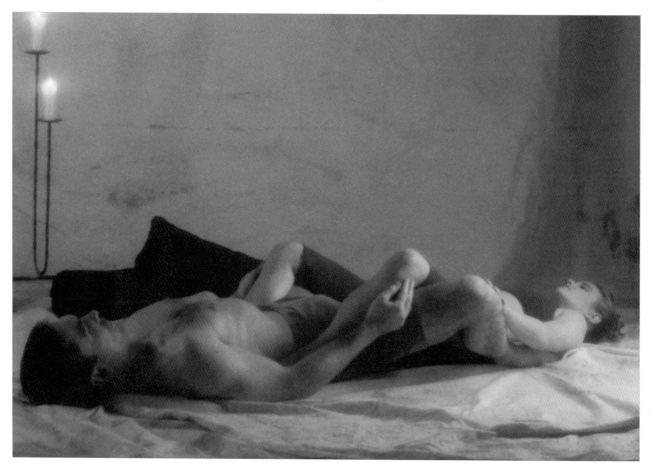

1. Both partners lie with their spines flat on the floor and their legs entwined; the supporting partner presses down with their legs on the other's inner thighs. The weight of the legs on the thighs will help to release any stiffness in the pelvic and groin areas.

2. (opposite) One partner sits up by taking their arms to their sides and pushing up. They then take hold of their partner's waist.

3. The reclining partner takes their arms out to the side and levers up into a sitting position.

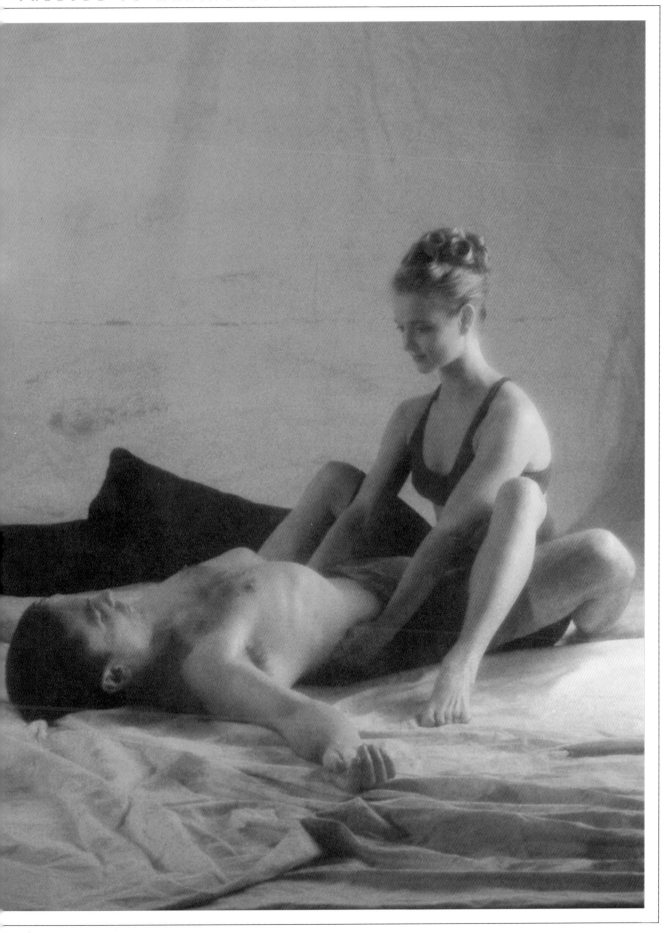

4. The couple support each other, lifting their lower backs and placing each other's heads first on the right shoulder and then on the left.

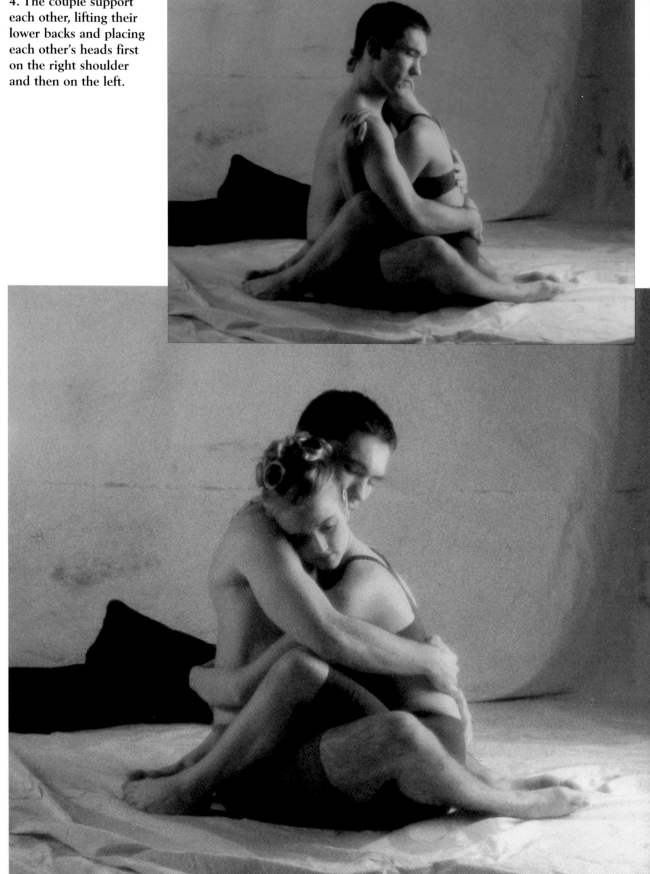

Rituals of lovemaking

T HE NURTURING, TOGETHERNESS, BALANCE and EMBRACE sequences are designed to prepare our minds and bodies for making love. However, far too often little thought is given to creating an environment that will inspire lovemaking. Such preparations are the rituals of lovemaking. Sexual rites and rituals exist in many ancient traditions. They help us achieve freedom from ourselves by surrendering to the experience of lovemaking and the interplay of energies between lovers.

Firstly, agree to set aside time for your lovemaking. In our busy, modern lives this is difficult to do, but it is important that both partners commit to a time to be together, preferably as far in advance as possible. You need to begin to tune into each other's energy by doing your yoga sequences or meditation together. Hindu texts advise that lovemaking is most potent between 7pm and midnight and again between midnight and 2am. Eat together at least an hour before making love, only light and easily digestible, wholesome food.

Secondly, you must create a sacred space. Choose a room and a time when you will be completely undisturbed. Tidy the space and use candles for a flattering and sensuous light. Provide pillows and cushions for support and ensure the room is warm enough to be unclothed in. Add colors that evoke the mood you want – reds, oranges, or purple for stimulation, dark blues and violets for relaxation, and green for healing.

Bathing in and burning scented oils adds a new dimension to your lovemaking. Essential oils, such as jasmine, rose, ylang-ylang or sandalwood, can soothe and stimulate both body and spirit.The potential for enhancing the eroticism of your lovemaking is unlimited. Try to use natural, organic materials as far as possible to create an atmosphere that pleases the spirit, uplifts the heart and elevates the mind.

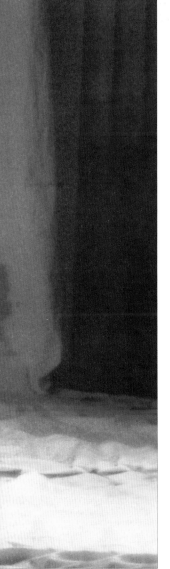

5. Both partners release from the position and lie back on the floor.

6. Switch positions so that the other partner's legs are on top, pressing down on the inner thighs, and repeat the sequence.

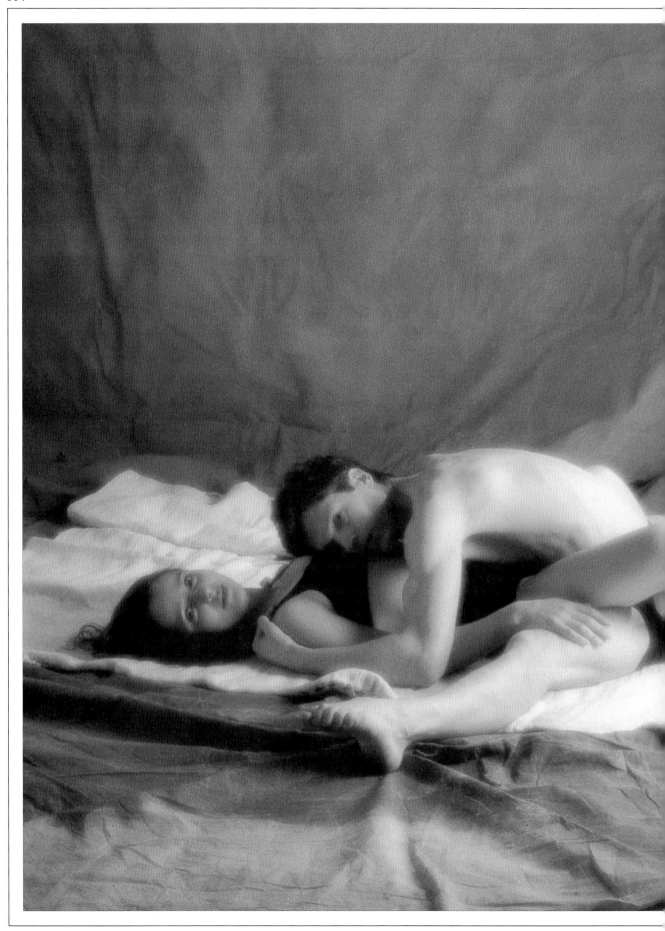

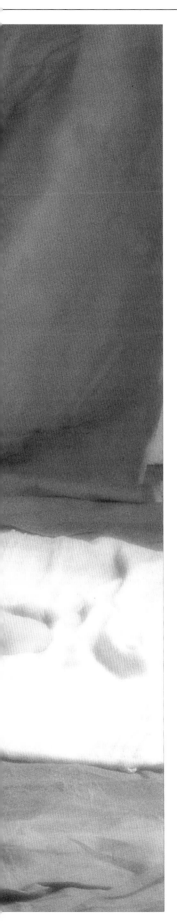

READY
FOR LOVE

The desire to learn about ourselves and others has long been expressed in the words of the ancient Greek Delphic oracle 'Know thyself'. It is the mainspring of all psychology. Such a wish, though, can never be fulfilled solely through knowledge of the ordinary kind, nor by reason alone. Even if we were to know a thousand times more than we already do, we would never reach bottom. We would still remain an enigma to ourselves. The only way to full knowledge lies in the act of love; this act is beyond thought, it transcends words. It is the daring plunge into the experience of union.

Be with each other, but do not possess each other. Possession is like grasping the wind. Togetherness comes of itself.

Beneath the universal, existential need for unity lies a more specifically psychological one: the desire for union between the masculine and feminine poles. Our state of polarization is most strikingly expressed in the myth that once man and woman were one, that later they were cut in half, and from then on each male has been seeking for the lost female part of himself in order to unite with her again – and vice versa.

Sexual polarization leads us to seek union in a specific, physical way: that of a joining with the opposite sex. The polarity between male and female principles exists also within each man and each woman. Just as physiologically man and woman each possess both sex hormones, they are also bisexual in the psychological sense. They carry in themselves the sense of receiving and of penetrating, of matter and of spirit.

The Art of Sensual Yoga works on all the physical, emotional and spiritual levels. It teaches us that love concerns making provision for another's physical comfort, learning about one another as sexual partners and, by experiment and fantasy, discovering what is pleasing to each other. On an emotional level it shows us that the affirmation of our own life, happiness, personal growth and freedom is rooted in our capacity to love, through which we learn care, respect and responsibility. Finally, on a spiritual level, *The Art of Sensual Yoga* is the road to self-knowledge through the act of love: a universal desire for union with another.

This final sequence has been developed to promote creative, playful loving. In many ways it is the culmination of all that has gone before, and yet, as will be experienced, it is much more than the sum of its parts.

1. UNION

PHYSICAL EFFECTS

This sequence will leave you feeling open, relaxed and ready for love. The standing positions at the beginning will help to ground the energy, and the leaning-back part of the sequence opens the lungs, leading to fuller expansion and thus allowing each partner to breathe more freely.

The next aspect of the sequence, the lying-down position, will, with the help of your partner, stretch the spine, the shoulders and the occipital, or back, area of the neck. Within this area there is often a build-up of uric acid and toxins, which can lead to tension. The stretching action here is excellent for eliminating tension in this area.

The body is now prepared for a more open and all-embracing stretch. Now there is a full extension of all the joints and muscles. It incorporates leg-opening, which releases and relaxes tension in the groin area, and a FORWARD BEND, which eases any tightness and accumulation of tension and strain in the lower back and kidneys.

Union is a long and continuous sequence of postures, encapsulating most of the different movements worked on throughout this book. It stretches the entire body and stimulates all the major organs. The spirit of the book is captured in Union as you work your way slowly through it: toning, releasing and then relaxing, finally, into the sensual and intimate postures at the end.

EMOTIONAL REFLECTIONS

There are eight major emotions: love and hatred; peace and anger; joy and sorrow; calmness and fear. This sequence exercises the physical areas that relate to these emotions.

Every organ in our body has an emotional aspect. For instance by working on the liver, which is the seat of anger, we can control our anger and create calm. Similarly, the heart is the seat of love; fear is related to the kidneys, and sadness, the lungs. By stretching in a way that stimulates these organs, we can control their negative aspects and promote the positive ones.

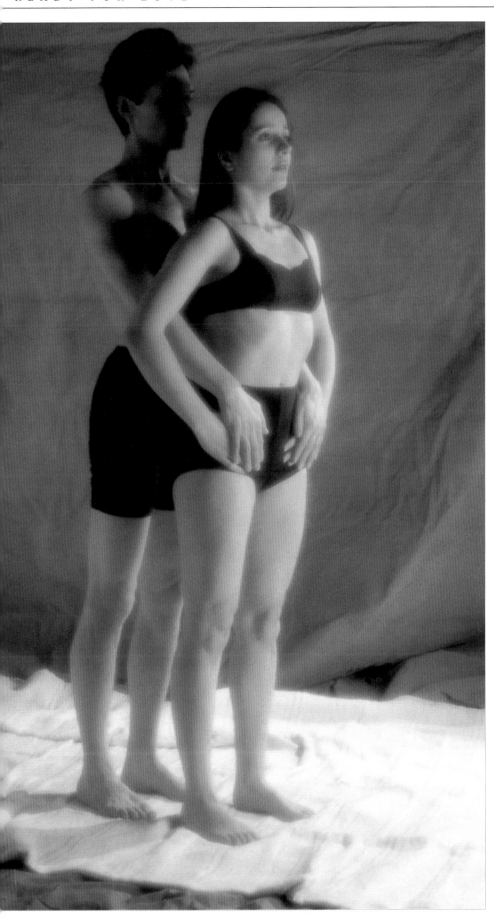

1. Stand one behind the other 1ft ($^1/_3$ meter) apart with feet firmly placed, rear partner's hands on the front one's pelvis, gently lifting. Stretch up through your legs, lift the kneecaps, keep the buttocks firm.

MEDITATION
We are filled with the power of creation

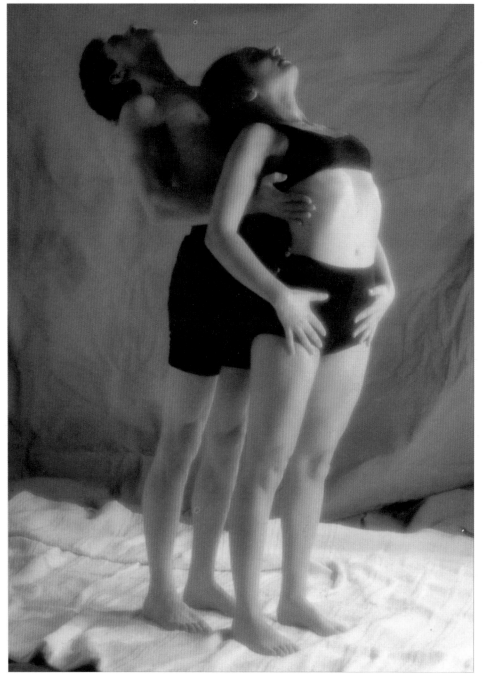

3. Then, keeping the hips in line with the heels, bend forward, the front partner folding their arms and sinking their whole body down towards the floor. The rear partner leans over, too, helping the front partner to extend down by placing their hand on the upper spine. Hold for four to five breaths.

4. Repeat 1–3, switching roles.

2. Stretch up and backwards, opening the chest, tucking in the shoulder-blades, lengthening the neck. The rear partner supports the front one's upper ribs. Hold for four to five breaths.

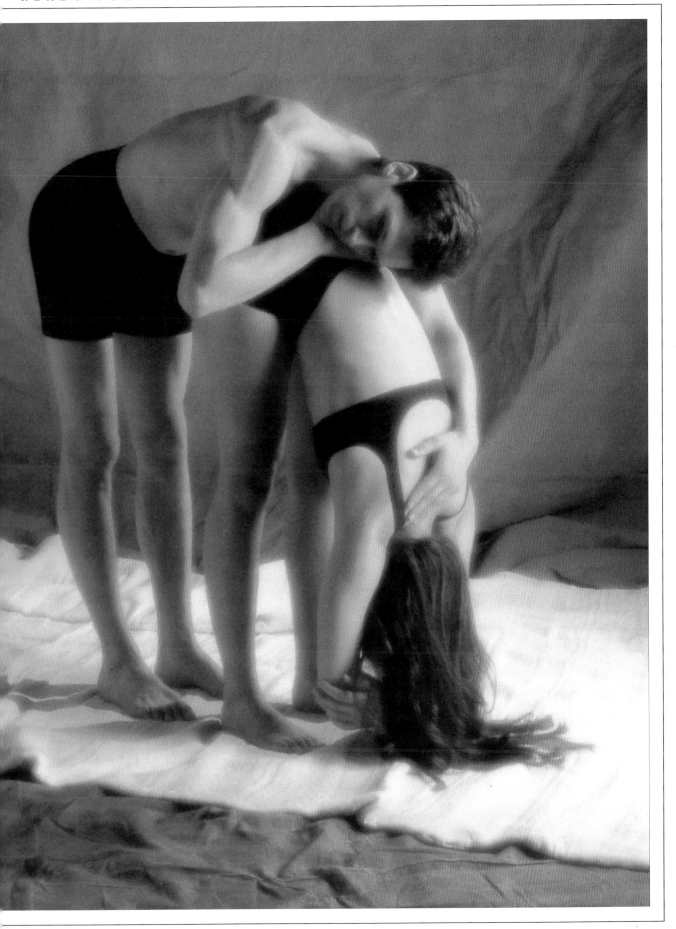

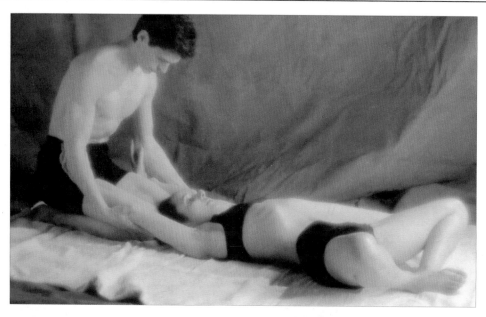

5. Lie down with the soles of the feet together and the heels in toward the groin. The rear partner sits on their heels at your head, holding your arms and giving you a firm backward stretch.

6. (below) Arch your back up. Allow your partner to place their hands under your shoulders and draw in your shoulder-blades to help you lift your upper chest. Hold for four to five breaths.

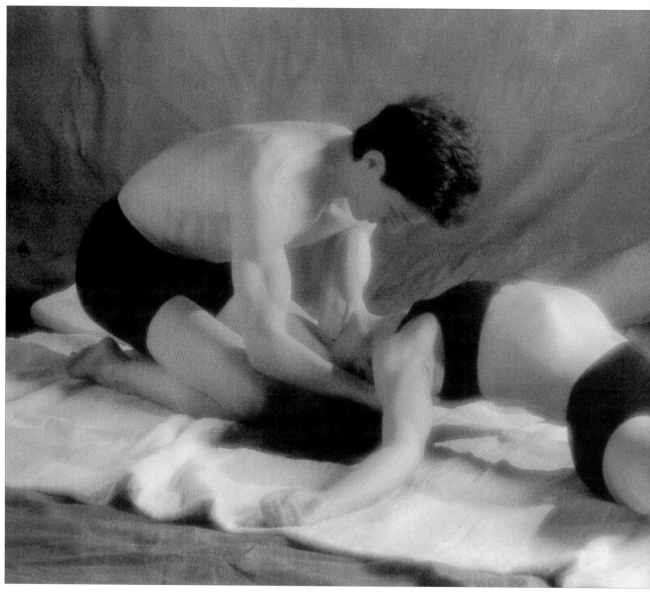

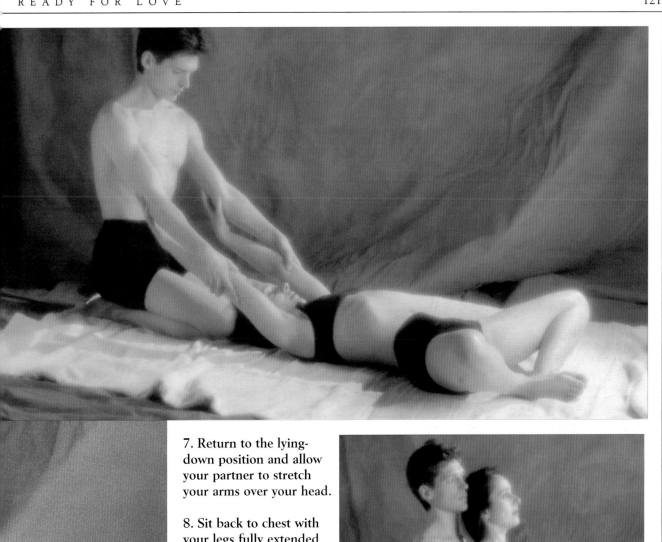

7. Return to the lying-down position and allow your partner to stretch your arms over your head.

8. Sit back to chest with your legs fully extended and wide apart. Your knees and toes are in an upward position, front partner's hips to rear's groin. Place your arms beside your hips and fully extend up through the spine, lifting the back ribs, keeping the shoulder-blades tucked in and collar-bones lifted, throat and jaw relaxed, eyes soft.

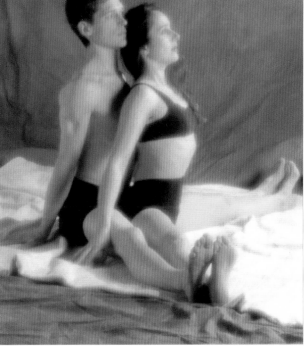

9. Twist towards the right leg. Keep the left leg firmly extended while you lift and turn more towards the right leg. Take the left hip forward and the right back. See if you can align the breastbone with your right leg, and, keeping the left buttock down, exhale and release down over your right leg. Hold this for four to five breaths.

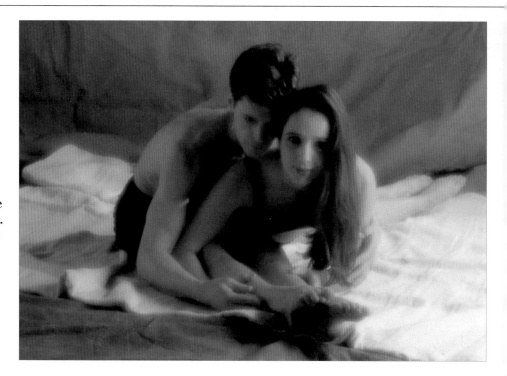

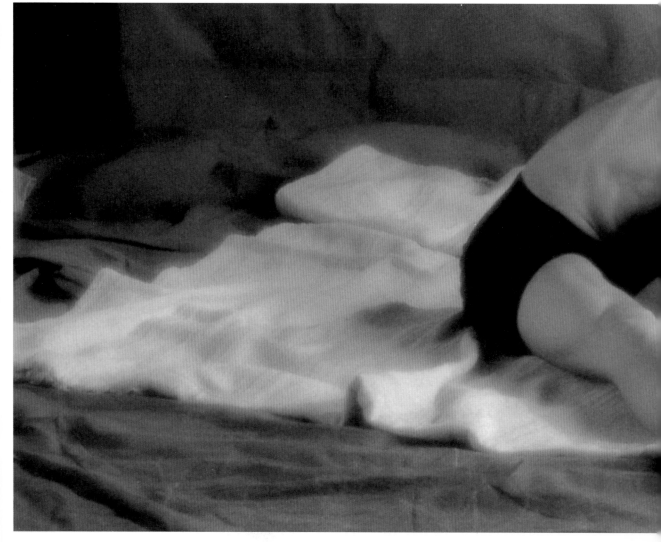

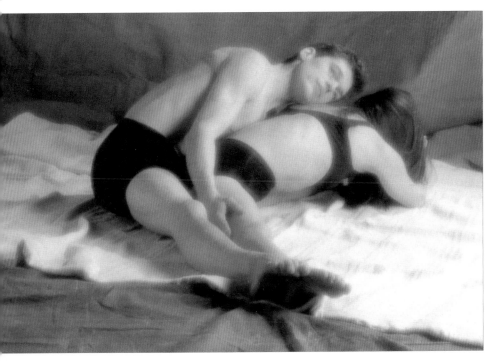

10. Lift up to the center, stretch up and then repeat on the other side. Hold for four to five breaths.

11. Come back to center and then both extend forward between the legs on an exhalation. The waist and chest extend forward. Hold for four to five breaths.

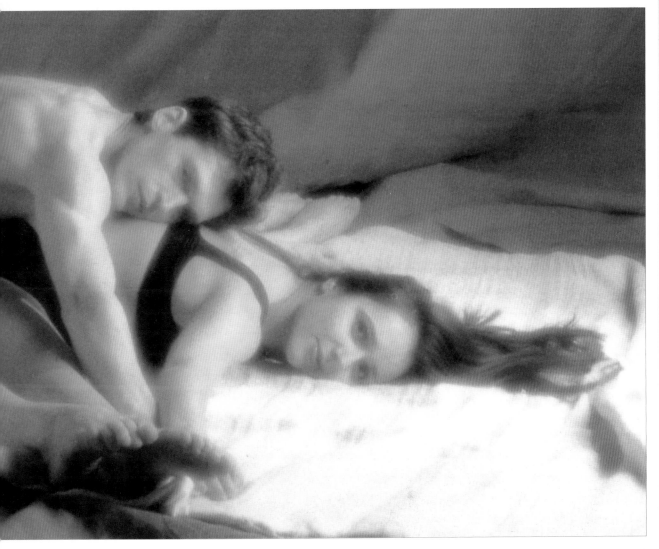

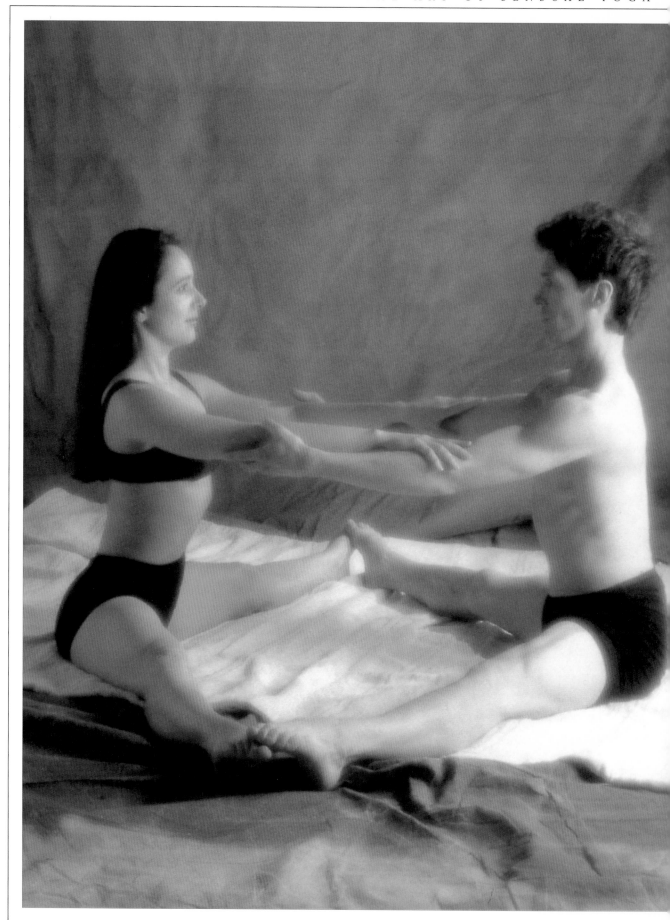

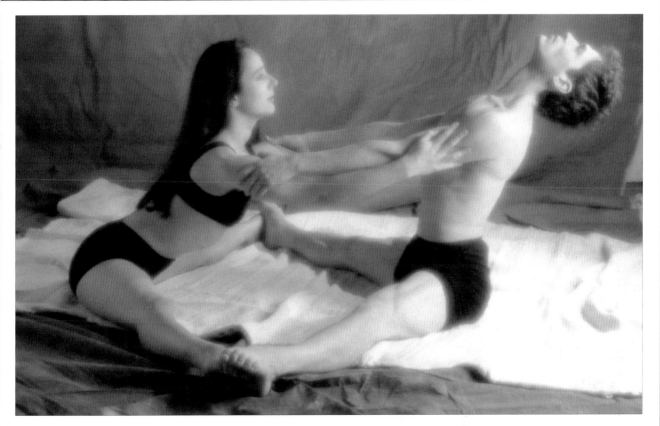

12. (opposite) Now sit
up facing each other,
with your legs wide
apart. Your arms are
extended in front of you,
each holding the other's
forearms. Focus on the
backs of your legs
extending into the floor,
shoulder-blades in and
chests lifting.

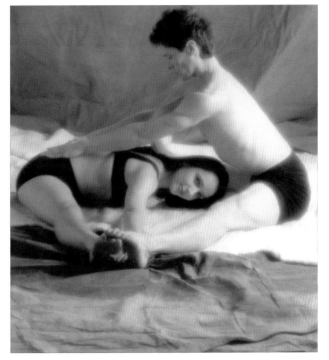

13. (above) On an
inhalation, one partner
leans back to open the
upper chest, while the
other leans forward,
supporting the upper
arms. The leaning-back
partner extends their
head back, pulls their
shoulder-blades in and
lifts their collar-bones.
Both hold for four to five
breaths.

14. Return to the center
and repeat the
movement with the other
partner leaning back.
Hold for four to
five breaths.

15. Come back up to the
center. One partner
leans into a forward
bend, lowering
themselves as far as they
can go, aided and
supported by the other

pressing on the spine.
Both partners should
keep their legs extended
and hold for four to five
breaths. Repeat with the
other partner leaning
forward.

16. Now one partner draws themselves in to the other, wrapping their legs around them while they are held around their waist. Arch back as your partner lifts your lower ribs. Keep the shoulder-blades in and extend your head back, while lifting your collarbones. Hold for four to five breaths.

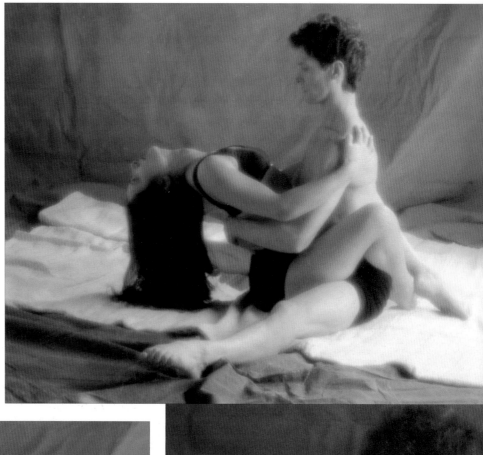

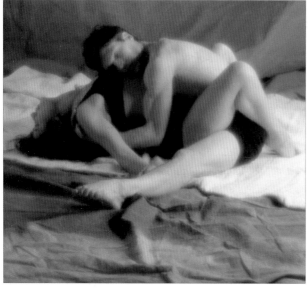

17. Still supporting your partner's back ribs slowly lower them to the floor with their back remaining arched, and their chest lifted. Lean forward and rest over your partner's chest, drawing their shoulderblades down. Hold for four to five breaths.

18. The lower partner then extends their spine and relaxes their neck. The upper partner stretches their trunk fully along the lower's abdomen. Hold for four to five breaths.

19. Repeat from 15–18, switching roles, then relax.

HELPFUL HINTS

• SEE IF YOU can follow the sequence through from the beginning to the end by going with the flow of the movements.

• TAKE TIME TO gain maximum benefit. Let the positions evolve in a relaxed way; don't try too hard. The important thing now is simply being together in the movements and achieving the best results you can without strain.

• IF THE FULL movement is not reached initially, don't be concerned. It will happen in time as *The Art of Sensual Yoga* becomes a part of your daily routine.

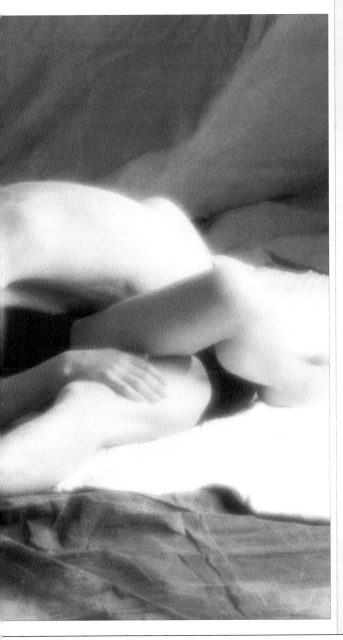

The new sex

Through the practice of *The Art of Sensual Yoga*, many couples with whom we have worked have come to understand that sex is not simply a pleasurable experience but our most creative force as well. It touches and inspires our lives and affects us emotionally, physically and spiritually. Some couples have gone on to explore Tantrism – the new sex – which provides a practical means of developing sexual union as a way of uniting body and mind.

The origins of Tantra are obscure but rooted in Hinduism. Its practice is based on four pillars of wisdom: yoga, yogic breathing, meditation and ritual. Central to Tantric philosophies is the the idea of a subtle form of energy that animates all forms of matter, including human beings. As discussed in chapter 5, in Tantric belief this energy, known as 'prana', flows through us all.

Yogic breathing teaches us how to control prana and store it in the body. Yoga in general instructs us on how to transform this life force into strength, vitality and nourishment for different parts of the body. Meditation helps, too, usually in the form of chanting, in which each sound is a kind of energy that has a unique vibrational quality, concentration on yantras – geometric designs that symbolize deities – or contemplation of mandalas – mystical diagrams that signify wholeness and totality, an expression of the psychological processes of unfolding and integration.

Tantric sex uses the act of making love, in combination with yogic positions, breathing, meditation and ritual to transform sexual energy into a vital, life-giving force that promotes health, well-being and, at its limits, permits an experience of the divine. It is an art through which we can experience our unlimited potential and the inherent divinity within each of us: the sacredness of sex. *The Art of Sensual Yoga*, then, is a gateway to ecstatic bliss. You need proceed no further, but if you do, let the art of Tantrism guide your way.

FURTHER EXPLORATIONS

The authors thoroughly recommend the following as further reading:

YOGA

B. S. Iyengar: *Light on Yoga* (Schocken,1987)
Sivananda Yoga Center: *Yoga Mind & Body* (Dorling Kindersley, 1996)

RELATIONSHIPS

Erich Fromm: *The Art of Loving* (Harper Collins,1996)
Michel Foucault: *The History of Sexuality*, 3 vols (Random House, 1990)
Ray Grigg: *The Tao of Relationships* (Humanics, 1988)

STRESS REDUCTION/MEDITATION

Paul Wilson: *Instant Calm* (Plume, 1995)

TANTRIC/TAOIST APPROACH TO SEXUAL RELATIONSHIPS

Mantak Chia and Maneewan Chia: *Healing Love through the Tao:
Cultivating Female Sexual Energy* (Healing Tao Books, 1986)
Mantak Chia and Maneewan Chia: *Taoist Secrets of Love: Cultivating
Male Sexual Energy* (Aurora Press, 1984)
Mantak Chia and Maneewan Chia: *Taoist Ways to Transform Stress into
Vitality* (Healing Tao Books, 1986)